OXFO

Series Editors

Kathy Boursicot

Reader in Medical Education and Deputy Head of the Centre for
Medical and Healthcare Education,
St George's, University of London

David Sales

Consultant in Medical Assessment

OXFORD ASSESS ~~AND~~ PROGRESS
your prescription for exam success

Written by clinicians and educational experts, these unique guides present complete coverage for your exam revision, with illustrative material and tips to help you suceed in your medical exams.

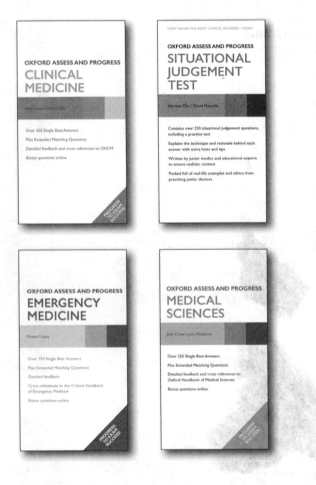

www.oup.com

OXFORD ASSESS AND PROGRESS

Clinical Specialties

Second Edition

Edited by

Luci Etheridge

Consultant Paediatrician and Senior Fellow in Clinical Leadership,
Barking, Havering and Redbridge University Hospitals NHS Trust

Alex Bonner

Specialist Trainee in Anaesthesia and Critical Care,
North West Deanery

OXFORD
UNIVERSITY PRESS

OXFORD
UNIVERSITY PRESS

Great Clarendon Street, Oxford, OX2 6DP,
United Kingdom

Oxford University Press is a department of the University of Oxford.
It furthers the University's objective of excellence in research, scholarship,
and education by publishing worldwide. Oxford is a registered trade mark of
Oxford University Press in the UK and in certain other countries

First Edition published 2010
Second Edition published 2013

Impression: 1

British Library Cataloguing in Publication Data
Data available

Library of Congress Cataloging in Publication Data
Library of Congress Control Number: 2012944655

ISBN 978-0-19-965758-2

Printed in China by
C & C Offset Printing Co. Ltd

Series Editor Preface

The Oxford Assess and Progress Series is a groundbreaking development in the extensive area of self-assessment texts available for medical students. The questions were specifically commissioned for the series, written by practising clinicians, extensively peer-reviewed by students and their teachers, and quality assured to ensure that the material is up to date, accurate, and in line with modern testing formats.

The series has a number of unique features, and is designed to be as much a formative learning resource as a self-assessment one. The questions are constructed to test the same clinical problem-solving skills that we use as practising clinicians, rather than only to test theoretical knowledge. These skills include:

- gathering and using data required for clinical judgement
- choosing the appropriate examination and investigations, and interpretation of the findings
- applying knowledge
- demonstrating diagnostic skills
- ability to evaluate undifferentiated material
- ability to prioritize
- making decisions and demonstrating a structured approach to decision making.

Each question is bedded in reality and is typically presented as a clinical scenario, the content of which has been chosen to reflect the common and important conditions that most doctors are likely to encounter both during their training and in exams! The aim of the series is to build the reader's confidence in recognizing important symptoms and signs and suggesting the most appropriate investigations and management, and in so doing to aid the development of a clear approach to patient management which can be transferred to the wards.

The content of the series has deliberately been pinned to the relevant *Oxford Handbook*, but in addition has been guided by a blueprint which reflects the themes identified in *Tomorrow's Doctors* and *Good Medical Practice* to include novel areas such as history taking, recognition of signs (including red flags), and professionalism.

Particular attention has been paid to giving learning points and constructive feedback on each question, using clear fact- or evidence-based explanations as to why the correct response is right and why the incorrect responses are less appropriate. The question editorials are clearly referenced to the relevant sections of the accompanying *Oxford Handbook* and/or more widely to medical literature or guidelines. They are designed to guide and motivate the reader, being multi-purpose in nature and covering, for example, exam technique, approaches to difficult subjects, and links between subjects.

Another unique aspect of the series is the element of competency progression from being a relatively inexperienced student to being a more experienced junior doctor. We have suggested the following four degrees of difficulty to reflect the level of training, so that the reader can monitor their own progress over time:

- graduate should know ★
- graduate nice to know ★ ★
- foundation doctor should know ★ ★ ★
- foundation doctor nice to know ★ ★ ★ ★

We advise the reader to attempt the questions in blocks as a way of testing their knowledge in a clinical context. The series can be treated as a dress rehearsal for life on the ward by using the material to hone clinical acumen and build confidence by encouraging a clear, consistent, and rational approach, proficiency in recognizing and evaluating symptoms and signs, making a rational differential diagnosis, and suggesting appropriate investigations and management.

Adopting such an approach can aid not only success in examinations, which really are designed to confirm learning, but also—more importantly—being a good doctor. In this way we can deliver high-quality and safe patient care by recognizing, understanding, and treating common problems, but at the same time remaining alert to the possibility of less likely but potentially catastrophic conditions.

David Sales and Kathy Boursicot, Series Editors

A Note on Single Best Answer and Extended Matching Questions

Single best answer questions are currently the format of choice being widely used by most undergraduate and postgraduate knowledge tests, and therefore most of the assessment questions in this book follow this format.

Briefly, the single best answer question presents a problem, usually a clinical scenario, before presenting the question itself and a list of five options. These consist of one correct answer and four incorrect options or 'distractors' from which the reader has to choose a response.

Extended matching questions, also known as extended matching items, were introduced as a more reliable way of testing knowledge. They are still widely used in many undergraduate and postgraduate knowledge tests, and are therefore included in this book.

An extended matching question is organized as one list of possible options followed by a set of items, usually clinical scenarios. The correct response to each item must be chosen from the list of options.

All of the questions in this book, which are typically based on an evaluation of symptoms, signs, or results of investigations either as single entities or in combination, are designed to test *reasoning* skills rather than straightforward recall of facts, and utilize cognitive processes similar to those used in clinical practice.

The peer-reviewed questions are written and edited in accordance with contemporary best assessment practice, and their content has been guided by a blueprint pinned to all areas of *Good Medical Practice*, which ensures comprehensive coverage.

The answers and their rationales are evidence-based and have been reviewed to ensure that they are absolutely correct. Incorrect options are selected as being plausible, and indeed they may appear correct to the less knowledgeable reader. When answering questions, the reader may wish to use the 'cover' test in which they read the scenario and the question but cover the options.

Kathy Boursicot and David Sales, Series Editors

Preface to the Second Edition

During the journey through medical school as a student, you experience medicine in a range of settings, from the rural general practice to the inner-city teaching hospital. You encounter doctors working in a wide range of specialties, many of which will be appealing future career choices and many of which will seem daunting. Specialty attachments may be the first time that you encounter people with mental illness, or children, or pregnant women. Trying to absorb all of these new experiences while also continuing to work towards final examinations can seem like a roller-coaster ride to some!

In partnership with the well-established *Oxford Handbook of Clinical Specialties*, the *Oxford Assess and Progress Clinical Specialties* volume seeks to tie together the clinical specialties and to provide a grounding in knowledge that may get pushed to the back burner when medicine and surgery have to be revised. This second edition has been produced in line with the new edition of the *Oxford Handbook of Clinical Specialties*, and builds on the success of the first book, bringing you questions on the latest hot topics, current issues, and core material. The questions in each chapter have been written by experienced doctors working within the specialty, who are familiar with the common presentations, pathologies, and dilemmas that are encountered. Their knowledge of teaching medical students about their specialty, often within the confines of very short attachments, has been transferred to these pages. All of the questions map on to medical school curricula and are rooted in real-life clinical encounters. The grading system allows you to judge for yourself which knowledge is core and which might require some further reading. We have added many new guidelines and key websites to guide this reading, and we hope that you will find these useful. The strong focus on clinical experiences also allows you to look forward to and prepare for your time as a foundation doctor.

We hope that, as a result of working through these questions, your interest in and appreciation and understanding of the different clinical specialties will grow, and you will have a useful tool for judging your own learning needs.

Luci Etheridge and Alex Bonner

Acknowledgements

The editors would like to thank all of the contributors for their hard work in combining their specialist knowledge with clinical experience to provide this resource of stimulating, realistic questions with considered explanations. Thank you also to all of the reviewers—students and specialists—for your much valued feedback. We hope that we have managed to address your suggestions in this new edition. Finally, heartfelt thanks to our partners—to Aaron Cue, for his support during a period of new additions to the family, and Amy Bonner, for tolerating the editing process, much of which occurred while living and working in Uganda.

Acknowledgements

Figure Acknowledgements

For Figures 2.1 and 2.6 and all of the figures in Chapter 7 on dermatology, we are grateful to Barts and the London NHS Trust for permission to reproduce their images, and to all of the patients who gave consent for images to be used.

Reproduced with permission from Oxford University Press: Plate 2.5: Collier *et al*, *Oxford Handbook of Clinical Specialties*, 9th edn, p. 132, Figure 1; Plate 4.1: Sundaram *et al*, *Training in Ophthalmology*, Figure 4.27; Plate 4.2: Sundaram *et al*, *Training in Ophthalmology*, Figure 7.19; Plate 4.3: Sundaram *et al*, *Training in Ophthalmology*, Figure 9.15; Plate 4.4: Sundaram *et al*, *Training in Ophthalmology*, Figure 5.51; Plate 4.5: Sundaram *et al*, *Training in Ophthalmology*, Figure 10.8; Plate 4.6: Sundaram *et al.*, *Training in Ophthalmology*, Figure 1.82; Plate 8.1: Hurley *et al*, *Oxford Handbook for the Foundation Programme*, 2nd edn, p. 187, Figure 5.

The Glasgow Coma Scale on pages 271 and 341 is reproduced from Teasdale G and Jennet B, 'Assessment of Coma and Impaired Consciousness: A Practical Scale', *The Lancet*, Vol. 304, 1974, with permission from Elsevier.

Finally, many thanks to all of the contributors who supplied images, and to their patients who gave consent for the images to be used.

Contents

Contents

About the Editors

Volume Editors

Luci Etheridge is a Consultant Paediatrician and Senior Fellow in Clinical Leadership at Barking, Havering and Redbridge University Hospitals NHS Trust in East London. She previously worked for four years with UCL Medical School, and was involved with the development of Fitness to Practise assessments for the General Medical Council and item writing for the Professional and Linguistics Assessments Board Part 1 and the Royal College of Paediatrics and Child Health. She is currently completing a doctorate in education at the Institute of Education, University of London.

Alex Bonner is a Senior Anaesthetic Trainee in the North West Deanery. He is regularly involved in the teaching of medical students, foundation doctors, and anaesthetic trainees who are preparing for their FRCA examinations. He is an instructor for Adult and Paediatric Advanced Life Support Courses, and has experience of practising anaesthesia and teaching in sub-Saharan Africa. He has also contributed to the development of Fitness to Practise assessments for the General Medical Council.

Series Editors

Katharine Boursicot is a Reader in Medical Education and Deputy Head of the Centre for Medical and Healthcare Education at St George's, University of London. Previously she was Head of Assessment at Barts and the London NHS Trust, and Associate Dean for Assessment at Cambridge University School of Clinical Medicine. She is consultant on assessment to several UK medical schools, medical Royal Colleges, and international institutions, as well as a consultant on the General Medical Council Professional and Linguistic Assessments Board Part 2 Panel and Fitness to Practise clinical skills testing.

David Sales is a general practitioner by training who has been involved in medical assessment for over 20 years, having previously been convenor of the MRCGP knowledge test. He has run item-writing workshops for a number of undergraduate medical schools and medical Royal Colleges, and internationally. He currently chairs the Professional and Linguistic Assessments Board Part 1 panel for the General Medical Council, and is their consultant on Fitness to Practise knowledge testing.

Contributors

Dr Erica Allason-Jones
NHS consultant in Genitourinary Medicine, Mortimer Market Centre (Camden PCT), London, UK

Professor Dinesh Bhugra
Professor of Mental Health and Cultural Diversity at the Institute of Psychiatry, King's College, London, and Honorary Consultant, Maudsley Hospital, London, UK

Dr Jennifer Birch
Consultant in Neonatal Medicine, Luton and Dunstable NHS Foundation Hospital Trust, Luton, UK

Dr Alex Bonner
Specialist Trainee in Anaesthesia and Critical Care, North West Deanery, UK

Dr Ruth Brown
Consultant in Emergency Medicine, St Mary's Hospital, Imperial College NHS Trust, and Honorary Senior Lecturer, Imperial College London, UK

Dr Will Coppola
Clinical Lecturer and Sub-Dean E-learning, UCL Medical School, London, UK, and salaried General Practitioner

Dr Jonathan Darling
Senior Lecturer in Paediatrics and Child Health, University of Leeds, and Honorary Consultant Paediatrician, Leeds Teaching Hospitals NHS Trust, Leeds, UK

Mr Nev Davies
Consultant in Trauma and Orthopaedics, Royal Berkshire Hospital, Reading, UK

Dr James Dawson
Registrar in Anaesthesia and Intensive Care, Trent Region, UK

Dr Philippa Edwards
Salaried General Practitioner, Portsmouth, UK

Dr Luci Etheridge
Consultant Paediatrician and Senior Fellow in Clinical Leadership, Barking, Havering and Redbridge University Hospitals NHS Trust, London, UK

Dr Kamila Hawthorne
General Practice Principal in Cardiff, and Sub Dean for Assessment, School of Medicine, Cardiff University, Cardiff, UK

Mr Kevin Hayes
Senior Lecturer and Consultant in Obstetrics and Gynaecology, St George's Hospital, London, UK

Dr Virginia Hubbard
Consultant Dermatologist, Homerton University Hospital, and Clinical Senior Lecturer, Barts and the London School of Medicine and Dentistry, UK

Dr Vikram Jha
Senior Lecturer in Medical Education, Leeds Institute of Medical Education, University of Leeds, and Honorary Consultant Obstetrician, Bradford Teaching Hospitals NHS Trust, UK

Dr Gill McGauley
Reader in Forensic Psychotherapy, St George's University of London, and Consultant in Forensic Psychotherapy, Broadmoor Hospital, West London Mental Health NHS Trust, UK

Dr Isabel McMullen
Specialty Registrar in Psychiatry, South London and Maudsley NHS Foundation Trust, UK

Dr Matthew Mathai
Consultant Paediatrician, Bradford Royal Infirmary, and Honorary Lecturer in Paediatrics and Child Health, University of Leeds, UK

Dr Zeryab Setna
Research Fellow in Medical Education, Leeds Institute of Medical Education, University of Leeds, Leeds, UK

Mr Venki Sundaram
Specialty Registrar in Ophthalmology, London Deanery, London, UK

Miss Philippa Tostevin
Senior Lecturer in Surgical Education, St George's University of London, and Honorary Consultant Otolaryngologist, St George's Hospital, London, UK

Normal and Average Values

Biochemistry: reference intervals

All laboratory discourse is probabilistic. Drugs may interfere with any chemical method; as these effects may be method dependent, it is difficult for us to be aware of all of the possibilities. If in doubt, discuss the issue with the laboratory.

Substance	Specimen	Normal value
Adrenocorticotrophic hormone	P	< 80 ng/L
Alanine aminotransferase	P	5–35 IU/L
Albumin	P†	35–50 g/L
Aldosterone	P*	100–500 pmol/L
Alkaline phosphatase	P†	30–150 IU/L (adults)
α-fetoprotein	S	< 10 kU/L
α-amylase	P	0–180 Somogyi units/dL
Angiotensin II	P*	5–35 pmol/L
Antidiuretic hormone	P	0.9–4.6 pmol/L
Aspartate transaminase	P	5–35 IU/L
β-HCG	S	M: < 10 mIU/mL; F (non-pregnant): < 25 mIU/mL; F (4 weeks pregnant): > 1000 mIU/mL
Bicarbonate	P†	24–30 mmol/L
Bilirubin	P	3–17 μmol/L (0.25–1.5 mg/100 mL)
Calcitonin	P	< 0.1 micrograms/L
Calcium (ionized)	P	1.0–1.25 mmol/L
Calcium (total)	P†	2.12–2.65 mmol/L
Chloride	P	95–105 mmol/L

Substance	Specimen	Normal value
Cholesterol‡	P	3.9–7.8 mmol/L
VLDL	P	0.128–0.645 mmol/L
LDL	P	1.55–4.4 mmol/L
HDL	P	0.9–1.93 mmol/L
Cortisol	P	a.m.: 450–700 nmol/L; midnight: 80–280 nmol/L
C-reactive protein (CRP)	S	< 10 mg/L
Creatine kinase	P	M: 25–195 IU/L; F:25–170 IU/L
Creatinine (related to lean body mass)	P‡	70–≤150 μmol/L
CSF glucose	CSF	> 2/3 of blood range
CSF protein	CSF	< 40 mg/dL
CSF white cells	CSF	< 5/mm³
Ferritin	P	12–200 micrograms/L
Folate	S	2.1 micrograms/L
Follicle-stimulating hormone (FSH)	P/S	Luteal: 2–8 U/L Ovulatory peak: 8–15 U/L Follicular phase, and M: 0.5–5 U/L Post-menopausal: < 30 U/L
Gamma-glutamyl transpeptidase	P	M: 11–51 IU/L; F: 7–33 IU/L
Glucose (fasting)	P	3.5–5 mmol/L
Glycated (glycosylated) haemoglobin	B	5–8%
Growth hormone	P	< 20 mU/L
Iron	S	M: 14–31 μmol/L; F: 11–30 μmol/L
Lactate dehydrogenase (LDH)	P	70–250 IU/L
Lead	B	< 1.8 mmol/L
Luteinizing hormone	P/S	Premenopausal: 3–13 U/L Follicular: 3–12 U/L Ovulatory peak: 20–80 U/L Luteal: 3–16 U/L Post-menopausal: < 30 U/L
Magnesium	P	0.75–1.05 mmol/L
Osmolality	P	278–305 mosmol/kg
Parathyroid hormone (PTH)	P	< 0.8–8.5 pmol/L
Phosphate (inorganic)	P	0.8–1.45 mmol/L

Substance	Specimen	Normal value
Potassium	P	3.5–5.0 mmol/L
Prolactin	P	M: < 450 U/L; F: < 600 U/L
Prostate-specific antigen	P	0–4 ng/mL
Protein (total)	P	60–80 g/L
Red cell folate	B	0.36–1.44 µmol/L (160–640 micrograms/L)
Renin (erect/recumbent)	P*	2.8–4.5/1.1–2.7 pmol/mL/hour
Sodium	P†	135–145 mmol/L
Thyroid-binding globulin (TBG)	P	7–17 mg/L
Thyroid-stimulating hormone (TSH) (normal range widens with age)	P	0.5–5.7 mU/L
Thyroxine (T4)	P	70–140 nmol/L
Thyroxine (free)	P	9–22 pmol/L
Total iron-binding capacity	S	54–75 µmol/L
Triglyceride	P	0.55–1.90 mmol/L
Tri-iodothyronine	P	1.2–3.0 nmol/L
Urea	P†	2.5–6.7 mmol/L
Urate	P†	M: 210–480 µmol/L; F: 150–390 µmol/L
Vitamin B$_{12}$	S	0.13–0.68 nmol/L (< 150 ng/L)

* The sample requires special handling. Contact the laboratory.
† Range is significantly different in pregnancy (see below).
‡ Desired upper limit of cholesterol level would be < 5 mmol/L.
Abbreviations: P, plasma (heparin bottle); S, serum (clotted; no anticoagulant); B, whole blood (edetic acid (EDTA) bottle); CSF, cerebrospinal fluid specimen; IU, International Unit; M, males; F, females; HDL, high-density lipoprotein; LDL, low-density lipoprotein; VLDL, very-low-density lipoprotein.

Arterial blood gases

pH	7.35–7.45
P_aCO_2	4.7–6.0 kPa
P_aO_2	< 10.6 kPa
Base excess	±2 mmol/L

Note: 7.6 mmHg = 1 kPa (atmospheric pressure ≈ 100 kPa).

Haematology: reference intervals

Measurement	Reference interval
White cell count (WCC)	$4.0–11.0 \times 10^9$/L
Red cell count	M: $4.5–6.5 \times 10^{12}$/L; F: $3.9–5.6 \times 10^{12}$/L
Haemoglobin	M: 13.5–18.0 g/dL; F: 11.5–16.0 g/dL
Packed red cell volume (PCV) or haematocrit	M: 0.4–0.54 l/L; F: 0.37–0.47 l/L
Mean cell volume (MCV)	76–96 fL
Mean cell haemoglobin (MCH)	27–32 pg
Mean cell haemoglobin concentration (MCHC)	30–36 g/dL
Neutrophil count	$2.0–7.5 \times 10^9$/L; 40–75% WCC
Lymphocyte count	$1.3–3.5 \times 10^9$/L; 20–45% WCC
Eosinophil count	$0.04–0.44 \times 10^9$/L; 1–6% WCC
Basophil count	$0.0–0.1 \times 10^9$/L; 0–1% WCC
Monocyte count	$0.2–0.8 \times 10^9$/L; 2–10% WCC
Platelet count	$150–400 \times 10^9$/L
Reticulocyte count	$25–100 \times 10^9$/L; 0.8–2.0%
Erythrocyte sedimentation rate	< 20 mm/hour (but depends on age; see OHCM 7th edn, p. 356)
Activated partial thromboplastin time (VIII, IX, XI, XII)	35–45 seconds
Prothrombin time	10–14 seconds

International normalized ratio (INR)	Clinical state (see OHCM, pp. 334–5)
2.0–3.0	Treatment of deep vein thrombosis (DVT), pulmonary emboli (treat for 3–6 months)
2.5–3.5	Embolism prophylaxis in atrial fibrillation (see OHCM, p. 335)
3.0–4.5	Recurrent DVT and pulmonary embolism; arterial disease including myocardial infarction; arterial grafts; cardiac prosthetic valves (if caged ball, aim for 4–4.9) and grafts

Plasma chemistry in pregnancy

	Non-pregnant		Trimester 1		Trimester 2		Trimester 3	
Centile	2.5	97.5	2.5	97.5	2.5	97.5	2.5	97.5
Na^+ (mmol/L)	138	146	135	141	132	140	133	141
Ca^{2+} (mmol/L)	2	2.6	2.3	2.5	2.2	2.2	2.2	2.5
Corrected*	2.3	2.6	2.25	2.57	2.3	2.5	2.3	2.59
Albumin (g/L)	44	50	39	49	36	44	33	41
Free T_4 (pmol/L)	9	23	10	24	9	19	7	17
Free T_3 (pmol/L)	4	9	4	8	4	7	3	5
TSH	0	4	0	1.6	1	1.8	7	7.3

*Calcium corrected for plasma albumin (see OHCM, p. 670).

Other plasma reference intervals (not analysed by trimester)

	Non-pregnant	Pregnant
Alkaline phosphatase (IU/L)	3–300	Up to 450*
Bicarbonate (mmol/L)	24–30	20–25
Creatinine (µmol/L)	70–150	24–68
Urea (mmol/L)	2.5–6.7	2–4.2
Urate (µmol/L)	150–390	100–270

*Occasionally very much higher in apparently normal pregnancies.

- C-reactive protein levels do not change much during pregnancy.
- TSH levels may be low in the first half of a normal pregnancy (suppressed by HCG). For other thyroid changes, see above and OHCS 9th edn, p. 25.
- Protein S levels fall during pregnancy, so protein S deficiency is difficult to diagnose.
- Activated protein C (APC) resistance is found in 40% of pregnancies, so special tests are required when looking for this. Genotyping for factor V Leiden and prothrombin G20210A is unaffected by pregnancy.

Paediatric reference intervals

Laboratories vary, so it is important to consult your own.

	Specimen	Normal value
Biochemistry (1 mmol = 1 mEq/L)		
Albumin	P	36–48 g/dL
Alkaline phosphatase	P	Depends on age*
α1-antitrypsin	P	1.3–3.4 g/dL
Ammonium	P	2–25 µmol/L; 3–35 micrograms/dL
Amylase	P	70–300 U/L
Aspartate aminotransferase	P	< 40 U/L
Bilirubin	P	2–16 µmol/L; 0.1–0.8 mg/dL
Bicarbonate	P	21–25 mmol/L
Calcium	P	2.25–2.75 mmol/L; 9–11 mg/dL
Neonates		1.72–2.47 mmol/L; 6.9–9.9 mg/dL
Chloride	P	98–105 mmol/L
Cholesterol	P, F	≤ 5.7 mmol/L; 100–200 mg/dL
Creatine kinase	P	< 80 U/L
Creatinine	P	25–115 µmol/L; 0.3–1.3 mg/dL
Glucose	F	2.5–5.3 mmol/L; 45–95 mg/dL (lower in newborn; fluoride tube)
IgA	S	0.8–4.5 g/L (low at birth, rising to adult level slowly)
IgG	S	5–18 g/L (high at birth, then falls, and finally rises slowly to adult level)
IgM	S	0.2–2.0 g/L (low at birth, rising to adult level by 1 year)
IgE	S	< 500 U/mL
Iron	S	9–36 µmol/L; 50–200 micrograms/dL
Lead	EDTA	< 1.75 µmol/L; < 36 micrograms/dL
Mg^{2+}	P	0.6–1.0 mmol/L
Osmolality	P	275–295 mosmol/L
Phenylalanine	P	0.04–0.21 mmol/L
Potassium (mean)	P	3.5–5.5 mmol/L
Protein	P	63–81 g/L; 6.3–8.1 g/dL
Sodium	P	136–145 mmol/L

Transferrin	S	2.5–4.5 g/L
Triglycerides	F, S	0.34–1.92 mmol/L (30–170 mg/dL)
Urate	P	0.12–0.36 mmol/L; 2–6 mg/dL
Urea	P	2.5–6.6 mmol/L; 15–40 mg/dL
Gamma-glutamyl transferase	P	< 20 U/L
Hormones: a guide (consult laboratory)		
Cortisol	P	9 a.m.: 200–700 nmol/L Midnight: < 140 nmol/L (mean)
Dehydroepiandrosterone sulphate	P	Days 5–11 of life: 0.8–2.8 μmol/L (range); 5–11 years: 0.1–3.6 μmol/L
17α-Hydroxyprogesterone	P	Days 5–11 of life: 1.6–7.5 nmol/L (range); 4–11 years: 0.4–4.2 nmol/L
T$_4$	P	60–135 nmol/L (not neonates)
TSH	P	< 5 mU/L (higher on days 1–4)

*Alkaline phosphatase (U/L): 0–0.5 years: 150–600; 0.5–2 years: 250–1000;
2–5 years: 250–850; 6–7 years: 250–1000; 8–9 years: 250–750; 10–11 years:
G = 259–950, B = ≤ 730; 12–13 years: G = 200–750, B = ≤ 785; 14–15 years:
G = 170–460, B = 170–970; 16–17 years: G = 75–270, B = 125–720; < 18 years:
G = 60–250, B = 50–200.
Abbreviations: B, boys; EDTA, edetic acid; F, fasting; G, girls; P, plasma; S, serum.

Haematology (mean ± ~1 standard deviation; range × 10^9/L (median in parentheses))

	Hb (g/dL)	MCV (fL)	MCHC (%)	Reticulocyte count (%)	White cell count	Neutrophil count	Eosinophil count	Lymphocyte count	Monocyte count
Days									
1	19.0 ± 2	119 ± 9	31.6 ± 2	3.2 ± 1	9–30	6–26 (11)	0.02–0.8	2–11	0.4–3.1
4	18.6 ± 2	114 ± 7	32.6 ± 2	1.8 ± 1	9–40				
5	17.6 ± 1	114 ± 9	30.9 ± 2	1.2 ± 0.2					
Weeks									
1–2	17.3 ± 2	112 ± 19	32.1 ± 3	0.5 ± 0.03	5–21	1.5–10 (5)	0.07–0.1	2–17	0.3–2.7
2–3	15.6 ± 3	111 ± 8	33.9 ± 2	0.8 ± 0.6	6–15	1–9.5 (4)	0.07–0.1	2–17	0.2–2.4
4–5	12.7 ± 2	101 ± 8	34.9 ± 2	0.9 ± 0.8	6–15	(4)		(6)	
6–7	12.0 ± 2	105 ± 12	33.8 ± 2	1.2 ± 0.7	6–15	(4)		(6)	
8–9	10.7 ± 1	93 ± 12	34.1 ± 2	1.8 ± 1	6–15	(4)		(6)	
Months (all the following Hb values are medians/lower limit for normal)									
3	11.5/9	88/88			6–15	(3)		(6)	
6	11.5/9	77/70			6–15	(3)		(6)	
12	11.5/9	78/72			6–15	(3)		(6)	
Years									
2	11.5/9	78/74			6–15	(3)		(5)	
4	12.2/10	80/75			6–15	(4)		(4)	

6	13/10.4	82/75			5–15	(4.2)		(3.8)
12	13.8/11	83/76			4–13	(4.9)		(3.1)
14B	14.2/12	84/77			4–13	(5)		(3)
14G	14/11.5							
16B	14.8/12	85/78	30–36	0.8–2	4–13	2–7.5 (5)	0.04–0.4	1.3–3.5	0.2–0.8
16G	14/11.5							
18B	15/13							

Note:
Basophil range: 0–0.1 × 10⁹/L; vitamin B12 (serum): ≥ 150 ng/L.

Basophil range: 0–0.1×10^9/L; vitamin B_{12} (serum): ≥ 150 ng/L.
Red cell folate (EDTA): 100–640 ng/mL.
Platelet counts do not vary with age: 150–400×10^9/L.
Abbreviations: B, boys; G, girls.

Abbreviations

ABC	Airway, breathing, circulation
ABCDE	Airway, breathing, circulation, disability, exposure
ADHD	Attention deficit hyperactivity disorder
ALS	Advanced Life Support
ASA	American Society of Anesthesiologists
ATLS	Advanced Trauma Life Support
AUDIT	Alcohol Use Disorders Identification Test
BMI	Body mass index
BP	Blood pressure
bpm	Beats per minute
C	Celsius
CD4+	Cluster of differentiation 4
cm	Centimetre
CNS	Central nervous system
CO	Carbon monoxide
CO_2	Carbon dioxide
COPD	Chronic obstructive pulmonary disease
CPAP	Continuous positive airway pressure
CPR	Cardiopulmonary resuscitation
CRP	C-reactive protein
CSF	Cerebrospinal fluid
CT	Computed tomography
CTG	Cardiotocography
CVP	Central venous pressure
DDH	Developmental dysplasia of the hip
DEXA	Dual-energy X-ray absorptiometry
dL	Decilitre
DMSA	Dimercaptosuccinic acid
DVLA	Driver and Vehicle Licensing Agency
ECG	Electrocardiogram
EEG	Electroencephalogram
ENT	Ear, nose, and throat
EOG	*Emergencies in Obstetrics and Gynaecology* (Oxford University Press)

ESR	Erythrocyte sedimentation rate
FSH	Follicle-stimulating hormone
FTA-ABS	Fluorescent treponemal antibody absorption test
GABA	Gamma-aminobutyric acid
GCS	Glasgow Coma Scale
GGT	Gamma-glutamyl transpeptidase
GI	Gastrointestinal
GMC	General Medical Council
GP	General practitioner
Hb	Haemoglobin
HBcAb	Hepatitis B virus core antibody
HBeAg	Hepatitis B virus e antigen
HBsAb	Hepatitis B virus surface antibody
HBsAg	Hepatitis B virus surface antigen
HBV	Hepatitis B virus
HCG	Human chorionic gonadotropin
Hg	Mercury
HIV	Human immunodeficiency virus
HPV	Human papillomavirus
HRT	Hormone replacement therapy
Hz	Hertz
Ig	Immunoglobulin
IM	Intramuscular
INR	International normalized ratio
IUD	Intrauterine device
IUS	Intrauterine system
IV	Intravenous
IVF	*In-vitro* fertilization
kg	Kilogram
L	Litre
LH	Luteinizing hormone
LPA	Lasting Power of Attorney
m	Metre
MAOI	Monoamine oxidase inhibitor
MAST	Military antishock trousers
MCHC	Mean corpuscular haemoglobin concentration
MCNS	Minimal change nephrotic syndrome
MCV	Mean corpuscular volume

MEWS	Modified Early Warning Score
MI	Myocardial infarction
mL	Millilitre
mm	Millimetre
mmol	Millimole
mph	Miles per hour
MRI	Magnetic resonance imaging
mU	Milli-units
NICE	National Institute for Health and Clinical Excellence
NSAID	Non-steroidal anti-inflammatory drug
O_2	Oxygen
OHCS	*Oxford Handbook of Clinical Specialties*
ORT	Oral rehydration therapy
P_aCO_2	Partial pressure of carbon dioxide in arterial blood
P_aO_2	Partial pressure of oxygen in arterial blood
pCO_2	Partial pressure of carbon dioxide
PCP	*Pneumocystis carinii* pneumonia
PEP	Post-exposure prophylaxis
PO	Per os (by mouth)
pO_2	Partial pressure of oxygen
RPR	Rapid plasma reagin
SIGN	Scottish Intercollegiate Guidelines Network
SLE	Systemic lupus erythematosus
SSRI	Selective serotonin reuptake inhibitor
THR	Total hip replacement
TPPA	*Treponema pallidum* particle agglutination
TURP	Transurethral resection of the prostate
U	Unit
UTI	Urinary tract infection
VDRL	Venereal Disease Research Laboratory
VF	Ventricular fibrillation
VT	Ventricular tachycardia
WHO	World Health Organization
ZIG	Zoster immunoglobulin

How to use this book

Oxford Assess and Progress, Clinical Specialties has been carefully designed to ensure you get the most out of your revision and are prepared for your exams. Here is a brief guide to some of the features and learning tools.

Organization of content

Chapter editorials will help you unpick tricky subjects, and when it's late at night and you need something to remind you why you're doing this, you'll find words of encouragement!

Chapters begin with **single best answer (SBAs)** questions followed by **Extended Matching Questions (EMQs)** questions. Answers can be found at the end of each chapter beginning with the SBA answers, and then the EMQ answers.

How to read an answer

Unlike other revision guides on the market, this one is crammed full of feedback, so you should understand exactly why each answer is correct, and gain an insight into the common pitfalls. With every answer there is an explanation of why that particular choice is the most appropriate. For some questions there is additional explanation of why the distracters are less suitable. Where relevant you will also be directed to sources of further information, such as the *Oxford Handbook of Clinical Specialties*, websites, and journal articles.

→ www.bmj.com/cgi/content/full/334/7583/35?grp = 1

Progression points

The questions in every chapter are ordered by level of difficulty and competence, indicated by the following symbols:

★   *Graduate 'should know'*—you should be aiming to get most of these correct.

★★   *Graduate 'nice to know'*—these are a bit tougher but not above your capabilities.

★★★   *Foundation Doctor 'should know'*—these will really test your understanding.

★★★★ *Foundation Doctor 'nice to know'*—give these a go when you're ready to challenge yourself.

Oxford Handbook of Clinical Specialties

The OHCS page references are given with the answers to some questions (e.g. OHCS 9th edn → p. 340). Please note that this reference is the **ninth edition** of the OHCS, and that subsequent editions are unlikely to have the same material in exactly the same place.

Chapter 1

Obstetrics and gynaecology, and genitourinary medicine

*Zeryab Setna, Erica Allason-Jones,
Kevin Hayes, and Vikram Jha*

This chapter will be of interest and help to all those studying the health-care of women. Obstetrics and gynaecology, like all fields of medicine, continues to evolve at a rapid pace, and keeping up to date with the latest literature, guidelines, and protocols can be a daunting task. In the follow-ing questions we have tried to encompass all of the important areas of this subject.

Pregnancy can be a joyful experience for both the mother and her family. However, it can occasionally be associated with complications, resulting in severe short- and long-term harm to both the mother and her baby. This chapter covers the most important aspects of pregnancy and its commonly associated problems.

Gynaecological practices are changing constantly, with more empha-sis on management in primary care, conservative rather than surgical management of conditions, and an increase in sub-specialization, such as gynaecological oncology and urogynaecology. This chapter reflects these changes and covers the most common areas in this interesting field.

Sexual health is a specialty in its own right. The numbers of cases of sexually transmitted infections are rising in the UK, despite efforts to raise awareness of safe sex, so knowledge of their presentations is important. The UK also has the highest rate of teenage pregnancy in Europe, and the Government has set targets to improve access to contraceptive advice for women. In recent years, astounding advances have been made in the treatment of human immunodeficiency virus (HIV) infection, and people with HIV can now expect to have a much better quality of life.

Zeryab Setna

QUESTIONS

Single Best Answers

1. An 18-year-old woman who is 34 weeks pregnant has abdominal pain and moderate fresh vaginal bleeding. The symphysio-fundal height measures 41 cm and the uterus feels tense and tender. The patient's pulse rate is 98 bpm and her blood pressure is 90/50 mmHg. Which is the single most likely diagnosis? ★

A Cervical ectropion

B Placental abruption

C Placenta praevia

D Pre-term labour

E Vasa praevia

2. A 22-year-old woman comes to the antenatal booking clinic at 12 weeks' gestation. Which is the single most appropriate group of booking investigations? ★

A Full blood count, blood group, and hepatitis C serology

B Full blood count, blood group, and Venereal Disease Research Laboratory (VDRL) test

C Full blood count, thalassaemia screen, and thyroid function test

D Full blood count, thalassaemia screen, and urea and electrolytes

E Full blood count, thyroid function test, and VDRL test

3. A 20-year-old woman and her 23-year-old husband have been trying to conceive for 6 months without success. Her periods are regular. Which is the single most appropriate management? ★

A Arrange a semen analysis for the husband

B Arrange a laparoscopy and dye test for the woman

C Arrange luteal-phase progesterone levels for the woman

D Arrange referral to the assisted-conception unit for *in-vitro* fertilization (IVF)

E Reassure the couple and suggest that they keep trying

4. A 55-year-old woman has hot flushes. Her last period was 2 years ago. She is keen to start hormone replacement therapy (HRT). Which is the single most appropriate question to ask her before commencing HRT? ★

A Do any of your relatives have Alzheimer's disease?

B Do you know whether you have osteoporosis?

C Have any of your relatives suffered from premature menopause?

D Have you ever suffered from deep vein thrombosis?

E Have you ever suffered from depression?

5. A 34-year-old primiparous woman is having generalized tonic–clonic convulsions. She is 32 weeks pregnant. Her blood pressure on arrival is 150/110 mmHg, she has 3+ proteinuria, and she is still having convulsions. The fetal heart rate is reassuring. Which is the single most appropriate management? ★

A Diazepam and plan delivery

B Diazepam plus antihypertensive drug, and plan delivery

C Magnesium sulphate

D Magnesium sulphate plus antihypertensive drug

E Magnesium sulphate plus antihypertensive drug, and plan delivery

6. A 23-year-old woman is 34 weeks pregnant and has raised blood pressure. She is on 200 mg labetalol twice daily. Her blood pressure is 160/105 mmHg and she has 3+ proteinuria. She feels well, with no headaches or epigastric pain. The cardiotocograph (CTG) is reassuring. All blood tests are normal. Which is the single most appropriate management? ★

A Admit her to hospital for urgent delivery

B Admit her to hospital to stabilize her blood pressure

C Arrange for her to attend the day unit for twice-daily CTG

D Increase the labetalol dose, and follow up with the community midwife

E Increase the labetalol dose, and follow up in the day unit

7. A 14-year-old girl requests emergency contraception. She had unprotected intercourse with her 14-year-old boyfriend 2 days ago. She appears to understand the nature of emergency contraception. Which is the single most appropriate management? ★

A Advise her that she cannot have emergency contraception, as it is too long since intercourse took place

B Advise her that she is too young to be legally prescribed emergency contraception

C Prescribe emergency hormonal contraception and advise her about future contraception

D Prescribe emergency hormonal contraception only after informing her parents

E Prescribe emergency hormonal contraception only after informing social services

8. A 31-year-old woman has vulval soreness and recurrent white vaginal discharge. Microscopy shows the presence of hyphae. Which is the single most appropriate treatment option? ★

A Clindamycin

B Clotrimazole

C Doxycycline

D Erythromycin

E Metronidazole

9. A 35-year-old woman who is taking Cerazette® (a progestogen-only contraceptive pill) has a chest infection and is prescribed amoxicillin. Which single piece of advice should be given about her contraception? ★

A No additional contraceptive precautions are required

B Use additional precautions for the duration of the antibiotic course

C Use additional precautions for the duration of the antibiotic course and for 2 days after the end of the course

D Use additional precautions for the duration of the antibiotic course and for 7 days after the end of the course

E Use additional precautions for the remainder of the current packet of Cerazette®

10. A 32-year-old primipara is seen at 42 weeks' gestation. She is keen to go into labour naturally and refuses an induction of labour. Which is the single best reason to give for allowing induction of labour when counselling her? ★

A There is an increased risk of Caesarean section beyond 42 weeks' gestation

B There is an increased risk of intrauterine growth restriction beyond 42 weeks' gestation

C There is an increased risk of placental abruption beyond 42 weeks' gestation

D There is an increased risk of shoulder dystocia beyond 42 weeks' gestation

E There is an increased risk of unexplained fetal death beyond 42 weeks' gestation

11. The midwife on the delivery suite calls for help. A woman who has just had a normal delivery with active management of the third stage of labour is bleeding heavily. The bleeding started 15 minutes after delivery of the placenta. Her estimated blood loss is 900 mL. Her pulse rate is 95 bpm and her blood pressure is 100/55 mmHg. Which is the single most appropriate first-line management? ★

A Massage the uterus and give IM carboprost (Haemabate®)

B Massage the uterus and give IM Syntocinon

C Massage the uterus and start a Syntocinon infusion

D Massage the uterus and start a blood transfusion

E Take the woman to theatre immediately for examination under anaesthesia

12. A 32-year-old woman has increasing white vaginal discharge. She is 7 weeks pregnant. Her *Chlamydia* swab is positive. All other tests are normal. Which is the single most appropriate treatment? ★

A Amoxicillin

B Clindamycin

C Doxycycline

D Erythromycin

E Metronidazole

13. A 42-year-old woman has frequency, urgency, and urge incontinence. Examination is unremarkable and a midstream specimen
of urine is sterile. She is treated empirically for detrusor overactivity with
oxybutynin. Which is the single mechanism of action for this drug? ★

A Anti-adrenergic

B Anti-GABAergic

C Antimuscarinic

D Antinicotinic

E Antiserotonergic

14. A 60-year-old woman is recovering post-operatively following a vaginal hysterectomy and anterior vaginal repair. She has
had voiding difficulty and has been catheterized for 3 days. A catheter
specimen of urine is taken due to a low-grade pyrexia, and it confirms the
presence of a urinary tract infection (UTI). Which single organism is most
likely to be causative? ★

A *Escherichia coli*

B *Klebsiella pneumoniae*

C *Proteus* species

D *Pseudomonas* species

E *Staphylococcus epidermidis*

15. A 24-year-old woman has had an abnormal vaginal discharge
for the past week. It is off-white and non-itchy, with an offensive
odour. She has had one sexual partner in the last 8 months, and he has
no symptoms. There is an off-white vaginal discharge of pH 6.4 pooling in
the posterior fornix, with no inflammation of the vulva or vagina. Which
is the single most likely finding on a Gram-stained sample of the vaginal
discharge? ★

A Gram-negative intracellular diplococci

B Gram-positive and Gram-negative mixed bacteria

C Numerous lactobacilli

D Polymorphonuclear leucocytes

E Yeast cells with hyphae

16. A 24-year-old woman has regular painful uterine contractions at 26 weeks' gestation. She is 2 cm dilated. Her membranes are intact. The cardiotocograph (CTG) is reassuring. Which is the single most appropriate management plan? ★

A Admit her and administer analgesics and Syntocinon

B Admit her and administer antibiotics and intramuscular steroids

C Admit her and administer antibiotics and tocolytic drugs

D Admit her and administer tocolytic drugs and intramuscular steroids

E Reassure her and send her home

17. A 14-year-old girl has been sexually active for 6 months and seeks sexual health advice. She has a regular partner and has no symptoms. She is very anxious that her mother does not find out that she is sexually active, and wants reassurance that her confidentiality will be maintained. In which single situation might breaching her confidentiality be justified? ★

A She is found to have a sexually transmitted infection

B She is in a sexually abusive relationship

C She requests a prescription for the oral contraceptive pill

D She requests a termination of pregnancy

E None of the above, as she has an absolute right to confidentiality

18. A 25-year-old woman has her first routine cervical cytology test as part of the NHS Cervical Screening Programme. This shows 'mild dyskaryosis, CIN 1', and she is advised to have a repeat smear performed in 6 months' time. She has had the same sexual partner for 18 months and they both tested negative for sexually transmitted infections at the start of the relationship. She has a body mass index (BMI) of 30 kg/m² and uses a progestogen-only oral contraceptive pill. She smokes 15 cigarettes daily and drinks approximately 25 units of alcohol per week. She wants to know if there is anything she can do that might help to reverse the abnormality. Which single action that she can be advised about is most likely to decrease her risk? ★

A Get vaccinated against human papillomavirus (HPV) infection

B Give up smoking cigarettes

C Reduce alcohol consumption

D Reduce body mass index

E Switch to an alternative contraceptive pill

19. A 24-year-old woman requests post-coital contraception. Her condom broke 36 hours ago, on day 7 of a regular 29-day cycle. This is her second condom accident in 2 months. She has tried the oral contraceptive pill, but stopped it 6 months ago because of concerns about weight gain. She is undecided about future contraceptive use. A pregnancy test is negative. Which is the single most effective form of post-coital contraception for her? ★

A A combined oral oestrogen/progestogen pill

B A progestogen-only pill

C Insertion of a copper-containing intrauterine device (IUD)

D Insertion of a progestogen-containing intrauterine system (IUS)

E No post-coital contraception is required

20. A 27-year-old man has had mild dysuria for 1 week. He has been having sex with his current girlfriend for 4 weeks, occasionally using condoms. She has no symptoms. He last had sex with his previous female partner 3 months ago. There is a slight mucoid discharge at the urethral meatus. Which single organism is the most likely cause? ★

A *Chlamydia trachomatis*

B *Mycoplasma hominis*

C *Neisseria gonorrhoeae*

D *Trichomonas vaginalis*

E *Ureaplasma urealyticum*

21. A 32-year-old man has a history of weight loss and general malaise. He takes an HIV test. The result is positive and his CD4 + count is 180 x 10⁶/L (12%) (normal range is 450–1600 x 10⁶/L). He is otherwise well. He does not feel ready to start antiretroviral therapy straight away, but is keen to stay well in the interim. For which single organism should he be offered primary prophylaxis? ★

A *Cryptococcus neoformans*

B *Mycobacterium avium intracellulare*

C *Mycobacterium tuberculosis*

D *Pneumocystis jirovecii*

E *Toxoplasma gondii*

22. A 19-year-old woman has had pain in her vulval area for 4 days. A photograph of the vulval lesion is shown in Plate 1.1 (see Colour Plate section). Which is the single most likely diagnosis? ★

A Behçet's disease

B Genital herpes

C Lichen sclerosis

D Syphilitic ulcer

E Vulval cancer

23. A 19-year-old woman has had pain in her vulval area for 4 days. A photograph of the vulval lesion is shown in Plate 1.1 (see Colour Plate section). Which is the single most appropriate initial management? ★ ★

A Perform a vulval biopsy

B Prescribe oral aciclovir

C Prescribe oral azithromycin

D Prescribe oral prednisolone

E Prescribe topical clobetasol (Dermovate®)

24. A 26-year-old primigravida is in advanced labour. Her labour has been augmented using Syntocinon, so a cardiotocograph (CTG) is performed. This is shown in Plate 1.2 (see Colour Plate section). Which is the single most appropriate management? ★ ★

A Perform urgent fetal blood sampling

B Perform an emergency Caesarean section

C Reassure the woman

D Stop the CTG recording

E Stop the Syntocinon infusion

25. A 29-year-old man from South Africa has collapsed at work. An eye witness gives a clear description of a convulsion. The man is drowsy, barely rousable, and unable to communicate. His wife states that she fears he may be HIV positive. His breathing becomes erratic, and artificial ventilation is being considered. In which single situation should an HIV test be carried out, given that he is unable to give informed consent? ★ ★

A At the request of his wife, as next of kin

B If knowledge of his HIV status would benefit his care

C Prior to admitting him to the Intensive Therapy Unit

D Prior to any invasive procedure being performed

E Prior to making the decision to ventilate

26. A 23-year-old woman has a large, 20-week-sized cystic mass on her ovary. She undergoes laparotomy and oophorectomy, and histology confirms that this is a benign mucinous cystadenoma. Which is the single most likely ovarian tissue of origin for this type of cyst? ★ ★

A Epithelial

B Follicular

C Germ cell

D Sex cord

E Stromal

27. A 22-year-old woman who is struggling to conceive has the following hormone profile, taken on day 6 of her cycle:

- Luteinizing hormone (LH): 12 IU/mL (normal pre-menopausal range, 3–13 IU/mL)
- Follicle-stimulating hormone (FSH): 4 IU/mL (normal range, 3–20 IU/ mL)
- Testosterone: 18 ng/dL (normal range, 6–86 ng/dL)

An ultrasound scan shows numerous peripheral ovarian follicles. Which single set of symptoms is she most likely to have? ★ ★

A Amenorrhoea and infertility

B Amenorrhoea and pelvic pain

C Oligomenorrhoea and facial hair

D Oligomenorrhoea and pelvic pain

E Oligomenorrhoea and temporal headaches

28. A 24-year-old man who has sex with men has read on the Internet that his sexual orientation puts him at risk of hepatitis B virus (HBV) infection. He is interested in being immunized. His hepatitis status results are as follows:

- Hepatitis B virus surface antigen (HBsAg) negative
- Hepatitis B virus core antibody (HBcAb) positive
- Hepatitis B virus surface antibody (HBsAb) negative
- Hepatitis B virus e antigen (HBeAg) negative

Which is the single most appropriate advice regarding his results and proposed immunization? ★ ★

A He has evidence of previous exposure to HBV and is a 'high-risk' carrier; immunization will not help

B He has evidence of previous exposure to HBV and is a 'low-risk' carrier; immunization will not help

C He has evidence of previous exposure to HBV with a partial immune response; immunization is unlikely to help

D He has evidence of previous exposure to HBV with an appropriate immune response; immunization is unnecessary

E He has no evidence of previous exposure to HBV, and should proceed with immunization as planned

29. A 16-year-old girl has had painful periods for 6 months. Her periods are regular and last 3 days. She misses a couple of days of school every month due to the pain. She is not sexually active. Which is the single most appropriate initial management? ★

A Combined oral contraceptive pill

B Gonadotrophin-releasing hormone analogues

C Intrauterine system (Mirena®)

D Mefenamic acid

E Tranexamic acid

30. A 36-year-old woman who is HIV positive discovers that she is pregnant. She is uncertain whether to continue the pregnancy, in particular because of the risk of the child acquiring her HIV infection. Her health is good and she has not yet needed to take antiretroviral therapy. If the pregnancy is managed appropriately, which is the single probability of her baby acquiring HIV infection? ★ ★

A 0% (i.e. no risk)

B Approximately 1%

C Approximately 15%

D Approximately 25%

E Approximately 40%

31. A 26-year-old woman with no children has had amenorrhoea for 6 weeks and has had some pelvic discomfort. Her pregnancy test is positive. Her pulse rate is 68 bpm and her blood pressure is 110/80 mmHg. An ultrasound scan shows an empty uterus, with normal adnexae. Her serum β-human chorionic gonadotrophin (β-HCG) level is 950 mIU/mL. Which is the single most appropriate next step in management? ★ ★

A Arrange for a laparoscopy

B Arrange for a laparotomy

C Repeat the β-HCG test after 48 hours

D Repeat the ultrasound scan and β-HCG test after 48 hours

E Repeat the ultrasound scan after 48 hours

32. A 32-year-old primiparous woman is 'small for dates' at 34 weeks' gestation. An ultrasound scan shows a singleton fetus with an abdominal circumference at the 10th centile. The amniotic fluid volume and umbilical artery Dopplers are normal. Which is the single most appropriate management? ★ ★

A CTG monitoring on alternate days

B Reassure her that the baby is growing appropriately

C Repeat the ultrasound scan in 2 weeks' time

D Repeat the ultrasound scan in 4 weeks' time

E Urgent delivery by Caesarean section

33. A 30-year-old nurse sustained a significant needle-stick injury during her last shift, 36 hours ago. The patient (i.e. 'donor') involved is HIV positive. He is taking antiretroviral therapy and his last viral load was 1000 copies/mL (acceptable load is < 5000 copies/mL). He is hepatitis B virus immune and negative for hepatitis C virus. The nurse also had unprotected sex earlier in her current menstrual cycle, and there is a possibility that she may be pregnant. Which is the single most appropriate advice regarding HIV post-exposure prophylaxis (PEP)? ★ ★

A It is already too late for her to start taking PEP

B PEP is contraindicated because of the possibility that she is pregnant

C She does not need PEP as the patient's viral load is so low

D She should start PEP without further delay

E The risks associated with PEP are higher than the risk of acquiring HIV

34. A 37-year-old woman is 15 weeks pregnant and requests a triple test to rule out Down's syndrome. Which is the single most appropriate advice to give her? ★ ★

A It is too early in pregnancy to have the triple test

B It is too late in pregnancy to have the triple test

C She could have the triple test arranged today

D She must first agree to have an amniocentesis if the test is screen positive

E The triple test will definitely be screen positive because of her age

35. A 42-year-old man attends a genitourinary medicine clinic and asks for a routine check for sexually transmitted infections. He has no symptoms and no abnormal clinical findings. Serological tests for syphilis show:

• Rapid plasma reagin (RPR) positive at a titre of 1:64
• *Treponema pallidum* particle agglutination (TPPA) assay positive
• Fluorescent treponemal antibody absorption test (FTA-ABS) positive

The same tests were negative 18 months ago. Which single stage of syphilis can be diagnosed? ★ ★

A Early latent

B Late latent

C Primary

D Secondary

E Tertiary

36. A 33-year-old woman has severe headache, blurred vision, abdominal pain, and bleeding per vaginum at 33 weeks' gestation. The fetal heartbeat is absent. Which is the single most important associated clinical sign that may help in diagnosis? ★ ★

A Brisk tendon reflexes

B Enlarged thyroid gland

C Oedema

D Raised jugular venous pressure

E Tachycardia

37. A 22-year-old woman is 6–8 weeks pregnant, and is brought into the Emergency Department in cardiac arrest. No other medical information about her is available. Which is the single most likely cause of her cardiac arrest in early pregnancy? ★ ★

A Miscarriage bleeding

B Pre-existing cardiac disease

C Pulmonary embolus

D Ruptured ectopic pregnancy

E Sepsis following termination of pregnancy

38. A 29-year-old gravid 2 + 1 woman is 35 + 6 weeks pregnant. She has a history of a previous Caesarean section. She has had regular uterine contractions for 4 hours and a per vaginum 'show'. Following speculum examination, which is the single most appropriate management? ★ ★

A CTG monitoring

B Fibronectin test

C IM steroid

D Rescue cerclage

E Tocolysis

39. A 22-year-old woman has acute onset of right iliac fossa pain but no vomiting. She has marked tenderness to palpation in the right iliac fossa. There is no rebound tenderness and some voluntary guarding. Her temperature is 37.2°C, her pulse rate is 80 bpm, and her blood pressure is 115/80 mmHg. Her pregnancy test is negative. An ultrasound scan shows a 7 cm right-sided haemorrhagic ovarian cyst with no free fluid. Which is the single most appropriate initial management? ★ ★ ★

A Admit her with a view to conservative management

B Allow her to go home, with advice to come back if the pain worsens

C Perform immediate laparoscopy in case the diagnosis is torsion

D Refer to the surgeons to rule out appendicitis

E Request a computed tomography (CT) scan to confirm the diagnosis

40. A 70-year-old woman has had vulval itching and discomfort for 12 months. There is widespread erythema on both labia minora extending on to the majora and involving the fourchette. There are no ulcers and there is no inguinal lymphadenopathy. Which is the single most appropriate initial management? ★ ★ ★

A Empirical treatment with potent corticosteroid ointment

B Immediate punch biopsy to exclude cancer

C Referral to the sexual health clinic to rule out sexually transmitted infection

D Treatment with oestrogen cream for atrophy

E Vulval excision to treat the affected area

41. A 24-year-old woman has dysmenorrhoea and deep dyspareunia. A transvaginal ultrasound scan shows a 4 cm endometrioma on the left ovary. The patient wants relief of her pain symptoms. She has also been trying to conceive for over 12 months. Which is the single most appropriate treatment to use? ★ ★ ★

A Combined oral contraceptive pill

B Danazol

C Gonadotrophin-releasing hormone analogues

D Laparoscopic surgery

E Medroxyprogesterone acetate (Provera®)

42. A previously well 67-year-old woman has abdominal distension, a large irregular pelvic mass, and ascites. An ultrasound scan, CT scan, and a raised CA125 confirm a likely ovarian carcinoma. Which is the single most appropriate first-line management? ★ ★ ★

A External beam radiotherapy

B High-dose progestogen therapy

C Hysterectomy, bilateral oophorectomy, omentectomy, and debulking

D Symptomatic palliative care

E Vincristine-containing chemotherapy

43. A 19-year-old woman is taking carbamazepine as treatment for her epilepsy. She is 16 weeks pregnant. She had been fit-free for 5 years before becoming pregnant, but has had two episodes of absence seizures in the past month. She has not informed the Driver and Vehicle Licensing Agency (DVLA) of her recent seizures. Which is the single most appropriate action to take at this stage? ★ ★ ★ ★

A Advise her to inform the DVLA immediately of her recent seizures

B Advise her to seek a second opinion about the safety of driving

C Inform the DVLA medical adviser immediately about the recent seizures

D Inform the patient's GP about the recent seizures

E Reassure the patient that there is no need to inform the DVLA

44. A 22-year-old primigravida undergoes a Neville-Barnes forceps delivery. The fetal head is delivered in the occiput posterior (OP) position. On examination the woman has a tear involving approximately one-third of the external anal sphincter thickness. What is the single most appropriate classification of this tear? ★ ★ ★ ★

A Second-degree tear

B Third-degree 3a tear

C Third-degree 3b tear

D Third-degree 3c tear

E Fourth-degree tear

Extended Matching Questions

Extended Matching Questions

Causes of testicular problems

For each patient, choose the *single* most appropriate management from the list of options below. Each option may be used once, more than once, or not at all. ★

A Antiviral drugs

B Arrange an ultrasound scan

C Aspiration

D Broad-spectrum antibiotics

E Doxycycline

F Emergency surgical referral

G Penicillin

H Reassurance

I Supportive treatment only

J Urgent urology referral

1. A 19-year-old man has had increasing scrotal pain for the last 24 hours. He has chills and general malaise. He had painful swellings in his neck and cheeks last week, but these are now improving. He has tenderness of the testis and epididymis on both sides. He has a regular girlfriend, who is well, and they always use condoms during sex.

2. A 17-year-old boy has sudden onset of severe pain in the left side of his scrotum, which came on 2 hours ago. He says that he has experienced a couple of similar but much milder episodes previously, but that these resolved very quickly. His scrotum is extremely tender on the left side. He has had a regular girlfriend for the last 6 months, who is well, and they use condoms for contraception.

3. A 26-year-old man has an intermittent swelling in the left side of his scrotum. He first noticed it a year ago, and it seems to come and go, being more noticeable when he stands up. It is not painful. When he stands up, there is an ill-defined mobile mass, which feels like a bag of worms, within the scrotum above the left testicle. He has had two sexual partners in the previous 3 months, but used a condom with only one of them.

4. A 24-year-old man has had increasing discomfort in his scrotum for the past 2 days, with some swelling on the right side. The left epididymis is easily palpable and tender, whereas on the right side both the epididymis and the testis are tender and slightly swollen. There is a small amount of mucoid discharge at the meatus. He started a new sexual relationship 4 weeks ago. His girlfriend is well and is taking the contraceptive pill.

5. A 31-year-old man has a gradual painless swelling of his right testicle. There is a firm lump in the testicle, with no associated tenderness. The lump does not transilluminate. He has been with his current girlfriend for over a year, and she is taking the contraceptive pill.

Causes of gynaecological neoplasia

For each clinical scenario, choose the *single* most likely diagnosis from the list of options below. Each option may be used once, more than once, or not at all. ★

A Cervical carcinoma

B Cervical ectropion

C Cervical intraepithelial neoplasia

D Choriocarcinoma

E Endometrial adenocarcinoma

F Endometrial adenoma

G Ovarian cystadenocarcinoma

H Ovarian cystadenoma

I Ovarian dermoid cyst

J Uterine leiomyoma

K Uterine leiomyosarcoma

L Vaginal carcinoma

M Vulval carcinoma

N Vulval intraepithelial neoplasia

O Vulval melanoma

6. A 38-year-old woman has progressive lower abdominal distension. She has a smooth pelvic abdominal mass that is palpable below the umbilicus. An ultrasound scan shows a 10 cm simple cystic right-sided mass and no ascites.

7. A 35-year-old para 4 woman has post-coital bleeding. She has a regular 28-day cycle and uses the combined oral contraceptive pill. Her last cervical smear, taken 2 years ago, was normal. She has a smooth, centrally red cervix with mild contact bleeding.

8. A 70-year-old woman has had recurrent vulval itching and soreness over the last 12 months that has failed to respond to topical steroid ointments. She has a 2 cm ulcerated lesion on the right labium majus.

9. A 30-year-old woman has heavy menstrual bleeding. Her periods are regular and there is no inter-menstrual or post-coital bleeding. Pelvic examination reveals that she has a bulky 10-week-sized uterus.

10. A 60-year-old nulliparous woman, who had her last menstrual period 4 years ago, has moderate post-menopausal bleeding. She is obese and has type 2 diabetes. Her last cervical smear, taken 12 months ago, was normal.

Causes of problems in early pregnancy

For each woman, choose the *single* most appropriate next investigation from the list of options below. Each option may be used once, more than once, or not at all. ★

A Amniocentesis

B β-Human chorionic gonadotrophin (β-HCG)

C Blood group and rhesus status

D Clotting screen

E Diagnostic laparoscopy

F Full blood count

G Glucose tolerance test

H Serum urea and electrolytes

I Transabdominal ultrasound scan

J Transvaginal ultrasound scan

K Urine for culture and sensitivity

L Urine pregnancy test

11. A 24-year-old primigravida is 10 weeks pregnant. She has frequency of micturition and some dysuria.

12. A 26-year-old primigravida is 10 weeks pregnant. She has marked abdominal tenderness and cervical excitation.

13. A 33-year-old woman is 14 weeks pregnant. She has vaginal bleeding. An ultrasound scan shows a 'snowstorm' appearance and no evidence of a fetus.

14. A 23-year-old woman is 7 weeks pregnant. She has been vomiting for the past 2 days. There is a moderate amount of ketones in her urine. Intrauterine pregnancy is confirmed by an ultrasound scan.

15. An 18-year-old woman has had amenorrhoea for 8 weeks, and now has nausea and feels generally unwell.

Urogynaecological disorders

For each clinical scenario, choose the *single* most likely diagnosis from the list of options below. Each option may be used once, more than once, or not at all. ★

A Bladder stone

B Congenital abnormality of the genitourinary tract

C Cystocele

D Detrusor overactivity

E Enterocele

F Genitourinary tract atrophy

G Genuine stress incontinence

H Interstitial cystitis

I Transitional-cell carcinoma of the bladder

J Rectocele

K Urethral stricture

L Urethritis

M Urinary tract infection

N Uterovaginal prolapse

16. A 60-year-old woman has a feeling of 'something coming down' in the vagina. She has no constipation or urinary symptoms. On examination, the cervix is visible on parting the labia.

17. A 60-year-old nulliparous woman has had urinary frequency and urgency for the last 6 months. She occasionally has small 'accidents' before she can get to the toilet.

18. A 16-year-old woman has had urinary incontinence almost continuously for a number of years, but has been too embarrassed to talk about it until now. She has a moist vulva and vagina and there is a central thin vaginal septum. There is no stress incontinence on coughing.

19. A 28-year-old woman has urinary frequency and dysuria. An endocervical swab is positive for *Chlamydia trachomatis*.

20. A 63-year-old woman has had urinary frequency, dysuria, and dyspareunia for the last 6 months. Her symptoms markedly improve on treatment with local oestradiol cream.

Causes of problems in pregnancy

For each patient, choose the *single* most likely diagnosis from the list of options below. Each option may be used once, more than once, or not at all. ★

A Asthma

B Deep vein thrombosis

C Eclampsia

D Epilepsy

E Essential hypertension

F Gestational diabetes

G Hypothyroidism

H Iron-deficiency anaemia

I Migraine

J Myocardial infarction

K Pancreatitis

L Pre-eclampsia

M Pulmonary embolism

N Thalassaemia

O Urinary tract infection

21. A 30-year-old unbooked primigravida has delivered a 4.7 kg baby at 36 weeks' gestation. There was difficulty in delivering the shoulders (shoulder dystocia).

22. An 18-year-old primigravida at 36 weeks' gestation has severe epigastric pain and headache. Her pulse rate is 80 bpm and her blood pressure is 140/98 mmHg. A urine dipstick test shows 2+ protein.

23. A 36-year-old para 4 woman is 35 weeks pregnant. She has sudden onset of shortness of breath. Her pulse rate is 100 bpm, her blood pressure is 100/70 mmHg, and her oxygen saturation is 94% on air. She recently had a sprained ankle, as a result of which her mobility has been restricted.

24. A 31-year-old para 6 woman books into the antenatal clinic. Her last delivery was 6 months ago. She feels tired and weak. She has a haemoglobin (Hb) level of 7.3 g/dL, a mean corpuscular volume (MCV) of 69 fL, and a mean cell Hb concentration (MCHC) of 30 g/dL.

25. A 25-year-old primigravida at 36 weeks' gestation has two episodes of tonic–clonic seizures and is confused. Her pulse rate is 78 bpm, her blood pressure is 110/70 mmHg, and her oxygen saturation is 98% on air. A urine dipstick test shows 3+ protein.

ANSWERS

Single Best Answers

1. B ★   OHCS 9th edn → p. 56

This woman is shocked. The abdominal pain and tense uterus suggest abruption. Blood loss may be concealed, so do not expect large amounts of visible bleeding. Placenta praevia is usually painless and the blood loss is greater, so is often noticed earlier. There are no contractions, so labour has not started, although delivery will be expedited as the patient is unwell. A cervical ectropion may bleed, but will not cause pain and shock.

2. B ★   OHCS 9th edn → p. 8

→ http://guidance.nice.org.uk/CG62/NICEGuidance/pdf/English

3. E ★   OHCS 9th edn → p. 292

Normal healthy couples can take up to a year to conceive, so investigations are not normally started until after 1 year of regular attempts to conceive.

4. D ★   OHCS 9th edn → p. 256

Overall, HRT doubles the risk of venous thromboembolism, so other risk factors need to be considered. HRT helps to reduce the risk of fractures in osteoporosis. There is no association with Alzheimer's disease; in fact, HRT may be protective. In some women, symptoms of depression may occur with some forms of HRT, but this would not be a contraindication.

→ www.rcog.org.uk/what-we-do/campaigning-and-opinions/briefings-and-qas-/rcog-and-hrt-debate

5. E ★   OHCS 9th edn → p. 49

Magnesium sulphate is the evidence-based treatment for eclamptic seizures. This patient also needs to have her blood pressure controlled carefully and delivery expedited.

→ www.rcog.org.uk/womens-health/clinical-guidance/management-severe-pre-eclampsiaeclampsia-green-top-10a

6. B ★   OHCS 9th edn → p. 48

Although the patient is currently asymptomatic, her blood pressure is above 160/100 mmHg and she has significant proteinuria, despite labetalol treatment. She needs admission for careful monitoring and controlled management with antihypertensives, and consideration of delivery if there is no improvement.

7. C ★   OHCS 9th edn → pp. 296–299

The girl appears to be Gillick competent, as she understands the nature of the treatment. Therefore she should be prescribed emergency contraception like any other patient. Emergency contraception can be given up to 72 hours after unprotected sex. Thought must be given to ongoing contraception to avoid further incidents.

→ www.dh.gov.uk/en/Publichealth/Healthimprovement/
Sexualhealth/Sexualhealthgeneralinformation/DH_4001998

8. B ★   OHCS 9th edn → p. 284

Hyphae indicate the presence of *Candida* or 'thrush'. Antibiotics are not appropriate treatment for a fungal infection. Clotrimazole is an antifungal topical treatment.

9. A ★   OHCS 9th edn → pp. 300–303

Most people remember that there is some interaction between the combined oral contraceptive pill and antibiotics. In truth, the evidence is slight, but the official advice to women taking the combined oral contraceptive pill is to use additional contraceptive methods for the duration of the course and for 7 oral-contraceptive-pill-taking days afterwards (i.e. the pill-free week does not 'count', so if a pill-free week is coming up, the woman might want to run two packets together). However, this rule does not apply to progestogen-only contraceptive pills, such as Cerazette®, and the woman should continue to take this continuously at the same time every day.

→ www.nhs.uk/Conditions/Combined-contraceptive-pill/Pages/
Interactionsother-medicines.aspx

10. E ★   OHCS 9th edn → pp. 54, 62

The reason why inductions are booked at 42 weeks is that the risk of intrauterine death increases significantly thereafter.

11. B ★ OHCS 9th edn → p. 84

Massaging the uterus helps to stimulate a contraction; the commonest cause is uterine atony. Syntocinon IM is the first-line treatment. It is a synthetic version of oxytocin and stimulates contractions. If bleeding does not stop, Syntocinon infusion and carboprost can be used along with other approaches for a major haemorrhage, such as blood transfusion and fresh frozen plasma. Blood loss of over 1000 mL, or clinical signs of shock, are considered to represent a major incident.

12. D ★ OHCS 9th edn → pp. 286–287

Amoxicillin, clindamycin, and metronidazole are ineffective against *Chlamydia*, and doxycycline is contraindicated in pregnancy.

13. C ★ OHCS 9th edn → p. 307

Detrusor contraction is activated via muscarinic cholinergic receptors, and oxybutynin is a direct antimuscarinic agent. Serotonin and noradrenaline (norepinephrine) are important for sympathetic activation, which reduces detrusor activity intrinsically. There are no nicotinic or GABAergic receptors in the bladder.

14. A ★

E. coli is by far the commonest cause of sporadic or catheter-related urinary tract infection. *Pseudomonas* species are usually only associated with prolonged catheterization, and *Staphylococcus epidermidis* is usually a contaminant.

15. B ★ OHCS 9th edn → p. 284

This is a description of bacterial vaginosis, which is caused by an altered vaginal flora and overgrowth of a number of different micro-organisms, which may show up on Gram staining.

16. D ★ OHCS 9th edn → p. 50

This woman has gone into premature labour, but this is at an early stage, so there is a possibility that it can be stopped with tocolytic drugs. However, steroids should still be given to mature the fetal lungs in case delivery goes ahead. There is no indication of infection, so antibiotics are not routinely given.

→ www.rcog.org.uk/womens-health/clinical-guidance/antenatal-corticosteroids-prevent-respiratory-distress-syndrome-gree

17. B ★   OHCS 9th edn → p. 297

The doctor has to judge whether the girl is Gillick competent, and if she is, she can consent to treatment herself. However, if she is thought to be the victim of any kind of sexual abuse and/or coercion, safeguarding rules trump her right of confidentiality, and the doctor has a duty of care to at least seek advice—for example, from the local named doctor for safeguarding children. The General Medical Council (GMC) gives guidance on this, which should be read.

→ www.gmc-uk.org/guidance/ethical_guidance/confidentiality.asp#29

18. B ★   OHCS 9th edn → pp. 272–273

All of these are protective against cervical changes. Human papillomavirus (HPV) vaccination has now been introduced into the UK and will help to prevent changes from occurring. However, in this case, in which the changes are already present, it will not be effective. The evidence shows that smoking is the most important risk factor in women who show mild change.

19. C ★   OHCS 9th edn → pp. 297–299

Combined oral contraceptive pills are no longer used for post-coital contraception. There is no efficacy advantage, and they have more side-effects than Levonelle® (a progestogen-only pill). Levonelle® may be an option. However, it does not offer the additional benefit of an ongoing method of contraception, and there is also a recognized failure rate. An IUD is always the most effective form of post-coital contraception for anyone, but in this case it has the added advantage of providing ongoing contraception (this is the patient's second condom accident in 2 months, and she cannot tolerate oral contraceptives). Mirena® coils are not used for post-coital contraception.

20. A ★

Chlamydia is the commonest sexually transmitted infection in the UK. Around 50% of men have no symptoms, but those that do may have dysuria, epididymo-orchitis, clear penile discharge, and low-grade fever.

21. D ★

Pneumocystis jirovecii (previously known as *Pneumocystis carinii*) can cause severe pneumonia (*Pneumocystis carinii* pneumonia or PCP) in immunocompromised individuals. The risk increases when the CD4+ count falls below $200 × 10^6$/L, especially if viral load is detectable. Therefore measures are taken to try to prevent this with antibiotic prophylaxis. It has been standard practice for many years to offer HIV patients with a CD4+ count of less than $200 × 10^6$/L primary prophylaxis against *Pneumocystis*.

Without prophylactic therapy, *Pneumocystis* is the single most likely serious or life-threatening opportunistic infection they will develop. Patients can develop *Cryptococcus neoformans* infection, but it is much less common, and primary prophylaxis is not given, although secondary prophylaxis would be continued in those who do develop it until their CD4+ count rises in response to therapy. *Mycobacterium avium intracellulare* is unlikely to be a problem with a CD4+ count of more than 100/µl, and primary prophylaxis is not routinely given. *Mycobacterium tuberculosis* can of course affect any patient regardless of CD4+ count, but primary prophylaxis is not given. *Toxoplasma gondii* is unlikely to be a problem with a CD4+ count of more than 50/µl, so primary prophylaxis would not be given in this case.

22. B ★   OHCS 9th edn → p. 268

Genital herpes causes multiple, painful sores on the vulva, and may also cause lymphadenopathy and flu-like symptoms. Behçet's syndrome can cause genital ulceration, but is rare. Lichen sclerosus causes white, atrophic-looking areas and usually occurs in older women. Syphilitic chancres are usually single and ulcerated.

23. B ★★   OHCS 9th edn → p. 268

This is herpes simplex virus infection, so antiviral treatment is required.

24. C ★★   OHCS 9th edn → pp. 44–45

This is a normal CTG, with a baseline of 110–160 bpm, a variability of more than 5 bpm, and accelerations seen.

25. B ★★

General principles of consent mean that the patient is the only person capable of giving consent for any investigation or treatment. If the medical information may guide his treatment (e.g. determining which drugs to start), investigations can be performed when he is unable to give consent. However, this is rarely straightforward, and the GMC guidance on consent should be read. Universal precautions mean that full infection control precautions should be taken for *all* patients, regardless of whether they are known to be HIV positive or not.

→ www.gmc-uk.org/guidance/ethical_guidance/consent_guidance_scope_of_treatment_in_emergencies.asp

26. A ★★   OHCS 9th edn → p. 281

Adenomata by definition are derived from the ovarian glandular epithelium.

27. **C** ★★ OHCS 9th edn → p. 252

A reversed LH:FSH ratio of around 3:1 and numerous small peripheral follicles in the ovaries are characteristic of polycystic ovarian syndrome. The symptoms of this include reduced periods, reduced fertility, hirsutism, acne, and weight gain.

28. **C** ★★

This patient has detectable HBcAb. The only way that an individual can develop core antibody is in response to hepatitis B virus infection. There is no core antigen in the vaccine. However, the patient is HBsAg negative and HBeAg negative, so he is not a chronic virus carrier. Unfortunately, he has not developed any HBsAb, which is the antibody that confers protective immunity (and what the vaccine aims to produce). There is some controversy as to whether vaccinating patients with a blunted response to previous hepatitis B virus infection achieves anything (if the infection did not result in immunity, the vaccine is unlikely to do any better). However, there is no evidence base for it.

29. **D** ★ OHCS 9th edn → p. 250

Mefenamic acid is effective for the management of period pain, and can be taken around the time of the period only. Tranexamic acid has some pain-relieving properties, but is more effective for the treatment of heavy periods. An IUS would be one option, but as the patient is not sexually active this would not be the first-line management. The pill may lighten periods, but does not necessarily relieve the pain. Gonadotrophin-releasing hormone analogues have no role.

30. **B** ★★ OHCS 9th edn → p. 23

The risks associated with modern management using antiretroviral drugs and elective Caesarean section are very low, although they are not eliminated completely.

31. **C** ★★ OHCS 9th edn → pp. 262–263

Although the history and empty uterus are suggestive of ectopic pregnancy, the β-HCG level is only slightly lower than 1000 mIU/mL. The woman is not shocked, so urgent treatment is not needed. β-HCG levels normally double over 48 hours, so a repeat test may confirm the diagnosis and allow decisions about management to be made. If the β-HCG concentration has not doubled, this is strongly suggestive of an ectopic pregnancy.

→ www.rcog.org.uk/womens-health/clinical-guidance/management-tubal-pregnancy-21-may-2004

32. C ★ ★   OHCS 9th edn → p. 52

Serial ultrasound scans to detect changes in abdominal circumference are accurate in diagnosing growth restriction. As this baby's abdominal circumference is less than the 10th centile, it may be growth restricted, and a scan should be repeated after 2 weeks.

→ www.rcog.org.uk/womens-health/investigation-and-management-small-gestational-age-fetus-green-top-31

33. D ★ ★

If the donor in a needle-stick injury is at high risk for blood-borne viruses, PEP should be started straight away until confirmatory testing can be done. Delays reduce the effectiveness. Many antiretroviral drugs are safe in pregnancy. Indeed, pregnant HIV-positive women are advised to take antiretroviral drugs to reduce the risk of HIV transmission to the fetus.

→ www.nice.org.uk/niceMedia/documents/pep.pdf

34. C ★ ★   OHCS 9th edn → pp. 10–11

The triple test measures maternal serum levels of α-fetoprotein, human chorionic gonadotrophin, and unconjugated oestriol. It uses these values, together with maternal age, to calculate the risk of certain conditions. It is a screening tool and is not diagnostic. If the risk is high, the mother can if she wishes choose further diagnostic tests.

35. A ★ ★

There are four stages of syphilis:

- Primary: characterized by painless ulcers, called chancres, at the site of infection. They may not be noticed. Chancres occur about 3 weeks after infection.
- Secondary: occurs 2–10 weeks after the chancres appear. Symptoms include a rash, mouth ulcers, lymphadenopathy, fever, and myalgia.
- Latent: occurs months to years after the initial infection if it goes untreated, and is usually asymptomatic, but the infection remains in the body.
- Tertiary: occurs years after initial infection in a minority of people, and can affect almost any part of the body.

Testing for syphilis can be complex because of the different stages. However, in an individual who is asymptomatic but has positive serological tests, this implies that the infection is latent. If the patient is known to have acquired the infection within the last 2 years, it is early latent. In this case, we can be completely confident that the infection is less than 2 years old, because we are told that the syphilis serology was negative 18 months ago.

36. A ★★   OHCS 9th edn → p. 48

These symptoms indicate severe pre-eclampsia. Brisk reflexes are commonly associated with pre-eclampsia. The others are just general clinical signs.

37. D ★★   OHCS 9th edn → pp. 262–263

The commonest cause of arrest and death in early pregnancy is hypovolaemia due to ruptured ectopic pregnancy, and it is the first consideration in a collapsed patient in early pregnancy. Heavy vaginal bleeding rarely presents in arrest, as help tends to be sought early for visible bleeding. The risk of pulmonary embolus is raised throughout pregnancy, but the most severe morbidity and mortality occur in later trimesters or post-partum, and both sepsis due to termination and pre-existing cardiac conditions are fortunately rare.

→ www.oaa-anaes.ac.uk/assets/_managed/editor/File/Reports/
2006–2008_CEMD_exec_summary.pdf

38. A ★★   OHCS 9th edn → p. 58

This woman may be in labour, and the single most appropriate plan of management in her case will involve a speculum examination and CTG to assess this. It is inappropriate to insert a cerclage at this gestation. A fibronectin test is contraindicated if there is PV bleeding. A single course of antenatal corticosteroids is administered to women between 24 + 0 and 34 + 6 weeks' gestation.

→ www.rcog.org.uk/files/rcog-corp/GTG%207.pdf,
→ www.rcog.org.uk/files/rcog-corp/GTG44PPROM28022011.pdf,
→ www.rcog.org.uk/files/rcog-corp/GTG1b26072011.pdf

39. A ★★★   OHCS 9th edn → p. 281

A patient with marked tenderness should not be allowed home. The history, examination, and ultrasound scan findings are highly suggestive, and are commensurate with a haemorrhagic cyst accident, which should be managed conservatively. The absence of vomiting, peritonism, and a pyrexia make torsion and appendicitis unlikely, and there is no need to refer the patient to the surgeons at this stage, as the diagnosis is basically straightforward. Therefore no further imaging is required at this stage.

40. A ★★★   OHCS 9th edn → p. 266

This is lichen sclerosus et atrophicus, a poorly understood inflammatory condition. It responds well to potent corticosteroid ointment, and biopsy is indicated if there is no response to treatment, or if an actual suspicious lesion such as an ulcer is present. Oestrogen cream is only effective for pure atrophy, and the likelihood of a sexually transmitted infection in a 70-year-old is very small. Excision is reserved for neoplastic conditions.

41. D ★★★   OHCS 9th edn → p. 288

All of the medical treatments listed are effective for pain, although there is increasing evidence that surgery gives the best results overall. Endometriomata tend to respond poorly to medical treatment, and usually require excision. Only surgical treatment has been demonstrated to improve subsequent fertility.

42. C ★★★   OHCS 9th edn → p. 283

Primary pelvic clearance and tumour debulking are the mainstays of ovarian cancer treatment initially. Neoadjuvant chemotherapy is a reasonable option in some women, but involves the use of carboplatin and paclitaxel, not vincristine. Hormonal treatment and radiotherapy have little or no place in ovarian cancer treatment, and palliative care is for women with terminal disease who have not responded to surgery and chemotherapy.

43. A ★★★★

Patients who have had a seizure should refrain from driving for 1 year. It is the patient's responsibility to inform the Driver and Vehicle Licensing Agency (DVLA), who may then seek information from the doctor. However, the doctor should inform the patient of this requirement, as they may be unaware of it.

→ www.epilepsysociety.org.uk/AboutEpilepsy/Livingwithepilepsy/ Drivingandtravel/Drivingandtransport

44. B ★★★★   OHCS 9th edn → p. 92

It is important to recognize and appropriately treat perineal tears in order to prevent future morbidity, particularly anal incontinence. Risk factors for tears include primiparity, large babies (> 4 kg), occiput posterior (OP) position, induction, epidural use, prolonged second stage, forceps use, and midline episiotomy.

Classification is as follows:

- first degree: injury to the perineal skin only
- second degree: injury to the perineum involving the perineal muscles but not the anal sphincter
- third degree: injury to the perineum involving the anal sphincter complex, consisting of the external anal sphincter (EAS) and internal anal sphincter (IAS):
- 3a: less than 50% of EAS thickness torn
- 3b: more than 50% of EAS thickness torn
- 3c: both EAS and IAS torn
- fourth degree: injury to the perineum involving the anal sphincter complex (EAS and IAS) and anal epithelium.

→ www.rcog.org.uk/files/rcog-corp/GTG2911022011.pdf

Extended Matching Questions

1. I ★

Although testicular pain should always be taken seriously, this young man has bilateral pain associated with fever and possible lymph node and parotid swelling. This suggests mumps. Although the treatment is supportive, the concern is about subfertility in post-pubertal men following mumps.

2. F ★

In contrast to the case in the previous question, this pain is severe and unilateral. The milder episodes may well have been caused by the testis retracting and twisting slightly in the past, but this severe episode suggests torsion, and the patient needs emergency surgical exploration to save the testicle.

3. H ★

This is a varicocele—that is, an enlargement of the veins that drain the testicle (the pampiniform plexus). It is similar to varicose veins in the leg. It tends to be more noticeable when standing, consistent with the effects of gravity. It is usually painless, but may be treated surgically if it is causing problems. There may be a small increased risk of infertility, but most men with varicoceles are not infertile.

4. E ★

Chlamydia is the commonest sexually transmitted infection, and causes epididymo-orchitis and urethral discharge. Gonorrhoea also causes discharge, but this is usually yellow and slimy, and dysuria is also prominent. Doxycycline or azithromycin are the usual first-line treatments for *Chlamydia*, but a diagnostic urine test should be sent first. Broad-spectrum antibiotics and most penicillins are not routinely used.

5. J ★

A firm, solid, painless testicular lump is considered to be a testicular tumour until proven otherwise, and should be referred to a urologist for diagnosis and treatment.

> *General feedback on 1–5:* When assessing testicular problems, differential diagnosis should include the following:
> - testicular torsion (acute, excruciatingly painful, and tender), which is a surgical emergency
> - tumour (a firm, painless, non-cystic lump)
> - epididymo-orchitis (discomfort and swelling, especially at the back of the scrotum, and possibly some discharge), which is usually caused by a sexually transmitted infection, such as *Chlamydia*, or by bacteria that cause urinary tract infections.
>
> Benign conditions include a varicocele, which does not usually cause any problems.

6. H ★

This is most likely as there are no clinical or ultrasound features of malignancy. The simple nature excludes a dermoid cyst, which is heterogeneous on scan.

7. B ★

This represents a large transformation zone (an area of squamous metaplasia), usually due to the high oestrogen levels observed in patients who are taking the combined oral contraceptive pill. It is physiological, but may cause post-coital bleeding and therefore concern.

8. M ★

This is commonly ulcerated and on the labia majora. Vulval intraepithelial neoplasia may be white and plaque-like but not ulcerated, and melanoma is usually pigmented.

9. J ★

These are very common and lead to uterine enlargement. If they occur inside the cavity, they can cause heavy periods.

10. E ★

Post-menopausal bleeding is assumed to be caused by endometrial adenocarcinoma until proven otherwise. This patient's age, obesity, and diabetes are also risk factors for endometrial adenocarcinoma. A normal smear 12 months previously makes cervical carcinoma less likely.

General feedback on 6–10: OHCS 9th edn → pp. 250, 266, 270, 278

11. K ★

Urinary tract infections are common in pregnancy, and these are typical symptoms.

12. J ★

This is likely to be an ectopic pregnancy, with abdominal pain and cervical excitation in the first trimester of pregnancy. A transvaginal ultrasound scan is the most sensitive way of confirming an empty uterus and looking at the Fallopian tubes to try to identify the pregnancy.

13. B ★

This woman is likely to have a molar pregnancy, or a hydatidiform mole. This is a rare occurrence caused either by only a placenta developing (i.e. with no fetus), or by a fetus with too many chromosomes developing with an abnormal placenta. The placenta produces large amounts of β-HCG, so this will indicate the diagnosis. The typical ultrasound appearance is of a 'snowstorm' uterus.

14. H ★

Hyperemesis gravidarum is severe morning sickness. Large amounts of vomiting can cause metabolic disturbance and may need to be treated with IV fluids.

15. L ★

The commonest cause of amenorrhoea is still pregnancy!

General feedback on 11–15: OHCS 9th edn → pp. 17, 260, 262

16. N ★

These are classical prolapse symptoms, for which a ring pessary may be a first-line solution. Lack of urinary and bowel symptoms makes anterior or posterior prolapse less likely.

17. D ★

Urgency and incontinence are most likely to represent detrusor overactivity.

18. B ★

Continuous leaking is suggestive of a bladder bypass. The patient's age and the presence of a congenital vaginal septum (40% coexistence with urinary abnormalities) suggests a congenital abnormality (e.g. an aberrant-ending ureter in the vagina).

19. L ★

Around 20–30% of women with *Chlamydia* infection have symptoms, which are often urinary. *Chlamydia* infects the anterior urethra and is described as urethritis (not a urinary tract infection).

20. F ★

The trigone is oestrogen sensitive, and atrophy can lead to urinary symptoms as well as vulvo-vaginal symptoms. A good response to local oestrogen cream is characteristic.

General feedback on 15–20: OHCS 9th edn → pp. 306–307

21. F ★

Gestational diabetes can go unrecognized, and leads to macrosomia and a large-for-dates baby, which can cause problems in vaginal delivery.

22. L ★

This is hypertension in pregnancy together with proteinuria, often with peripheral oedema. It can be asymptomatic—hence the need for blood pressure monitoring during pregnancy. However, headache and abdominal pain are symptoms that require further investigation and management.

23. M ★

The risk of pulmonary embolism is raised during pregnancy. Other risk factors here include the unexpected immobility. Pulmonary embolism causes pleuritic chest pain, shortness of breath, tachycardia, and hypoxia. It can be fatal, and therefore needs to be recognized and treated.

24. H ★

Anaemia is common in pregnancy because of the increased demand by the fetus and haemodilution by the increased plasma volume. Not all women need treatment. The World Health Organization (WHO) advises maintaining levels above 11 g/dL. However, this woman has a markedly decreased Hb level as well as symptoms of anaemia, namely tiredness. Her MCV and MCHC are low, indicating iron deficiency.

25. C ★

If left untreated, pre-eclampsia can progress and cause seizures. This is eclampsia. The low blood pressure here is post-ictal.

General feedback on 21–25: OHCS 9th edn → pp. 22, 24, 32, 48

Chapter 2

Paediatrics

Luci Etheridge, Jennifer Birch, Jonathan Darling, and Matthew Mathai

Children are not merely small adults. To be a good paediatrician requires as much knowledge about health as about disease. The normal patterns of growth and development can be a mystery to many, and paediatricians are often called upon to help to interpret these for confused parents. There is a unique need to be aware of the range of congenital disorders that may present before, at, or shortly after birth. Younger children cannot tell us their symptoms. Therefore paediatricians have to learn to pick up on non-verbal clues and often subtle signs, when the answer may lie in something unexpected and far removed from the traditional history and examination format. At the other end of the spectrum, adolescents have their own range of health issues and are traditionally an under-represented and often forgotten group. In this chapter, we aim to cover many of the key presentations and issues in children of all ages, from neonates to teenagers.

Even in this modern age, children are susceptible to infection. Respiratory and gastrointestinal infections are the commonest presentations in both general practice and paediatric hospital practice. Fortunately, most of these infections are self-limiting, but serious infections do occur and must be recognized. However, the leading cause of death in all children over 1 year of age is accidents. Recognizing risk factors for accidental and non-accidental harm is a major responsibility for all those working with children.

The questions in this chapter will test not only the common areas that present to paediatricians, but also relevant issues such as knowledge of disease factors, ethics, and risk management in relation to children and their families. However, the best way to learn about children is to get out there and meet them—play with them, talk to their parents and carers, and see them when they are ill and well. You will learn the most this way and be able to apply that knowledge and experience to answer questions such as these.

Luci Etheridge

QUESTIONS

Single Best Answers

1. A 1-day-old girl has a harsh systolic cardiac murmur all over the precordium with a thrill at the left sternal edge. Femoral pulses are palpable. A chest X-ray shows an enlarged heart, and an ECG shows left ventricular hypertrophy. Which is the single most likely diagnosis? ★

A Aortic stenosis

B Coarctation of the aorta

C Patent ductus arteriosus

D Pulmonary stenosis

E Ventricular septal defect

2. A 4-month-old boy is due to have his routine immunization. After the last set of immunizations, he had a 2 cm red area on his thigh around the injection site and seemed irritable for several hours. He has had a runny nose for the last 2 days but no fever. His mother asks whether it is all right to proceed with his immunizations. Which is the single most appropriate piece of advice to give? ★

A Postpone immunization until his runny nose has settled

B Immunize him in hospital

C Omit pertussis but proceed with the other immunizations

D Omit this set of immunizations

E Reassure the mother and proceed with the planned immunizations now

3. A 7-year-old girl is drowsy and panting, and has a capillary blood glucose level of 25 mmol/L and ketones and protein in her urine. Initial blood results show:

- sodium 145 mmol/L
- potassium 3.8 mmol/L
- creatinine 100 μmol/L
- urea 12 mmol/L
- calcium 2.6 mmol/L
- glucose 26 mmol/L.

She is given two fluid boluses of 10 mL/kg 0.9% saline, and is then started on a 0.9% saline infusion to deliver a total of maintenance plus 10% over 48 hours. IV insulin is also started. Two hours later she has improved, has passed urine, and is more alert. Her blood results show:

- sodium 143 mmol/L
- potassium 3.8 mmol/L
- creatinine 82 μmol/L
- urea 10 mmol/L
- calcium 2.2 mmol/L
- glucose 20 mmol/L.

Which single fluid should she now be given intravenously? ★

A 0.45% saline and 5% dextrose

B 0.45% saline and 5% dextrose with added calcium

C 0.45% saline and 5% dextrose with added potassium

D 0.9% saline

E 0.9% saline with added potassium

4. A 5-year-old girl had been passing hard stools once every 5 to 7 days for 6 months. She was started on two Movicol® Paediatric sachets daily. She continued this treatment for 1 month and started passing a stool every day, so her parents stopped it. For the last month she has been soiling her pants, with intermittent runny stools. She opens her bowels on the toilet most days, and passes pellet-like stools and an occasional large, hard stool. Which is the single main deficiency in her management so far? ★

A Colonoscopy should have been performed

B Glycerol suppositories should have been added

C Movicol® should have been continued for several more months

D She should have had an enema when she was first seen

E Stimulant laxatives should have been used

5. A 7-year-old boy wets the bed most nights and has never been reliably dry. He is a heavy sleeper. He has kept a star chart for 4 weeks and his parents have been supportive. His chart shows one dry night each week, with no particular pattern. He has a cub camp in 4 months' time. Urinalysis is negative. Which is the single most appropriate management? ★

A Star chart

B Enuresis alarm

C Desmopressin melts at night

D Imipramine tablets at night

E Oxybutynin tablets at night

6. A 1-year-old boy has had diarrhoea for the past 12 hours. At the beginning of the illness, he vomited twice. He has not passed urine for the past 6 hours. He is thirsty and restless, his eyes are sunken, the mucous membranes are dry, and skin turgor has decreased. His pulse rate is 160 bpm, and his capillary refill time is 2 seconds. Which is the single best description of his degree of dehydration and the appropriate initial fluid to give? ★

A Mild; oral rehydration solution

B Mild; 0.9% saline IV

C Moderate; oral rehydration solution

D Moderate; 0.9% saline IV

E Severe; 0.9% saline IV

7. A 20-hour-old term newborn boy has a short soft early systolic murmur on his baby check. He is pink, with no signs of respiratory distress, and has normally palpable femoral pulses and a normal apex beat. The murmur is heard at the upper left sternal edge, and radiates through the chest. There are no associated heaves or thrills. Which is the single most likely diagnosis? ★

A Atrial septal defect

B Innocent heart murmur

C Patent ductus arteriosus

D Pulmonary stenosis

E Ventricular septal defect

8. A 12-year-old girl, who recently arrived in the UK from South Asia, has had pain and swelling of both knees, ankles, and wrists for 5 days, and these symptoms come and go. Five weeks ago she had a cold and a sore throat. For the last day she has had a rash on her trunk, which has a pink border and is fading centrally. Both knees have an effusion and limited flexion to 70°. The girl's temperature is 39.2°C and her pulse rate is 160 bpm. Which single organism is likely to be responsible for this illness? ★

A *Corynebacterium diphtheriae*

B Human cytomegalovirus

C Epstein–Barr virus

D Group A β-haemolytic Streptococcus

E *Staphylococcus aureus*

9. A 6-year-old boy has had vomiting for 24 hours and has been unable to keep any liquids down, although he has not wanted to eat any food. Today he has central abdominal pain, which was coming and going but is now constant and sharp. He has pain when he tries to pass urine, and gets very upset if he is moved. He has opened his bowels once today and passed a loose stool. Which is the single most likely diagnosis? ★

A Appendicitis

B Gastro-oesophageal reflux

C Mesenteric adenitis

D Viral gastroenteritis

E Volvulus

10. A 39-week-gestation baby girl, who weighs 3.4 kg, is due for her baby check. She is lying supine. The examiner's left hand is stabilizing the pelvis and his right hand is grasping the left leg, flexed at the hip and knee, with his thumb over the lesser trochanter and the tip of his middle finger over the greater trochanter. He wants first to check whether the right hip is dislocatable with Barlow's manoeuvre. Which is the single most accurate description of how the examination should be performed? ★

A Adduct the leg to the midline and apply gentle anterior pressure over the greater trochanter

B Adduct the leg to the midline and apply gentle posterior pressure over the lesser trochanter

C Fully abduct the leg and apply gentle posterior pressure over the lesser trochanter

D Fully abduct the leg and apply gentle anterior pressure over the greater trochanter

E Partially abduct the leg and apply gentle anterior pressure over the greater trochanter

11. A 24-month-old girl enjoys 'feeding' her dolls. She does not like taking turns. She is able to walk upstairs with help but is unable to stand on one leg. She is able to scribble but is unable to draw a circle. She can say 'mama' and 'dada' with meaning, but no other recognizable words. In which single developmental area is she showing delay? ★

A Fine motor skills

B Gross motor skills

C Social skills

D Speech and language skills

E Play skills

12. A 14-year-old girl has chronic kidney disease. Her nephrologist advises that dialysis is the only option while she is awaiting renal transplant. She refuses to have dialysis, and appears to understand the consequence of not having treatment. She was in and out of local authority care between the ages of 1 and 6 years, but has been living with her parents for the last 8 years. Her mother, who has sole parental responsibility, wants her to have dialysis, but her father feels that she should decide for herself. The family have been through extensive counselling with the team, but have not been able to reach a consensus. Which single decision takes precedence when deciding further management? ★

A That of the father

B That of the local authority

C That of the mother

D That of the nephrologist

E That of the patient

13. A 2-month-old boy has faltering growth. He is a sweaty baby, particularly during breastfeeding. He has a palpable 4 cm liver edge. He is pale and has a respiratory rate of 60 breaths/minute, a heart rate of 180 bpm, and a blood pressure of 80/40 mmHg, and his oxygen saturation is 96% in air. His capillary refill time is 3 seconds, and his capillary blood glucose concentration is 5 mmol/L. Which single system of the body is most likely to be affected? ★

A Cardiovascular system

B Gastrointestinal system

C Metabolic system

D Neurological system

E Respiratory system

14. A 37-week-gestation baby who weighed 2.7 kg at birth is now 4 days old. He is being breastfed. During the first 24 hours of life he did not latch on to the breast well, and fed for approximately 5 minutes at a time every 4 to 5 hours. He is now feeding for 15–20 minutes every 2 to 3 hours. His weight today is 2.55 kg. His mother is worried about his weight loss. Which is the single most appropriate advice to give her? ★

A Any weight loss in the first week is worrying, and he should have supplementary feeds

B He has lost less than 10% of his birth weight, which is acceptable in the first week, and she should continue breastfeeding

C He has lost less than 10% of his birth weight, which is acceptable in the first week, but he should have supplementary feeds until he gains weight

D He has lost more than 10% of his birth weight, which is acceptable in the first week, and she should continue breastfeeding

E He has lost more than 10% of his birth weight, which is more than is normal in the first week, so he should have supplementary feeds

15. A 14-year-old Caucasian boy has had raised temperatures with drenching night sweats and malaise for 8 weeks. He has lost 4 kg in weight. He had a ventricular septal defect repaired in infancy. He looks pale, has extensive dental decay, and has small, linear areas of bleeding under his nail beds. He has a three-finger-breadth splenomegaly and a grade 2 systolic murmur, heard best in the lower left sternal edge. His temperature is 38°C. Which is the single most appropriate treatment? ★

A Antibiotics

B Chemotherapy

C Diuretics

D High-dose steroids

E Surgery

16. An 18-month-old African-Caribbean girl is not yet walking. She was breastfed for 9 months and is thriving along the 25th centile for weight. She has bow legs, Harrison's sulci, and swollen wrists. Which single vitamin deficiency is she most likely to have? ★

A Vitamin A

B Vitamin B_{12}

C Vitamin C

D Vitamin D

E Vitamin E

17. A mother brings her 7-month-old boy to the Emergency Department. She says he is always 'on the go', and that morning she saw him climb out of his cot and fall on to the laminate flooring, from a height of approximately 3 feet. He is now not moving his right leg. He has a spiral fracture of the right femur on X-ray. Which single part of the history will help most in deciding further management? ★

A Birth history

B Family medical history

C Developmental history

D Social history

E Systems review questioning

18. A 4-year-old Caucasian boy has poorly controlled asthma, despite being on a high-dose steroid inhaler and a leukotriene-receptor antagonist and compliant with his medication. He has recurrent chest infections and has significant nasal discharge. He also has poor growth, Harrison's sulci, and finger clubbing. Which is the single most appropriate next investigation? ★

A Bronchial brush biopsy

B Bronchoalveolar lavage

C CT scan of the chest

D Lung function tests

E Sweat test

19. A 4-year-old boy has periorbital oedema, central abdominal discomfort, and decreased urine output. His urine dipstick shows 3+ proteinuria and no blood. He is asthmatic, and recently had a bad 'cold.' Which is the single most likely diagnosis? ★

A Angioedema

B Nephrotic syndrome

C Post-streptococcal glomerulonephritis

D Postural proteinuria

E Systemic lupus erythematosus (SLE)

20. A 7-year-old boy with asthma has had a 'cold' and a temperature of 37.7°C for 24 hours. He has severe respiratory distress and requires 15 L/minute of oxygen to maintain his oxygen saturation above 95%. He is started on nebulized salbutamol therapy, which causes an initial improvement in his symptoms. He then suddenly deteriorates, with marked respiratory distress, hypoxia, and hypotension. Which is the single most likely diagnosis? ★

A Anaphylaxis

B Pleural effusion

C Pneumonia

D Pulmonary embolus

E Tension pneumothorax

21. A 6-year-old girl has had vomiting and central abdominal pain for 3 days. She has eczema and poorly controlled asthma. She looks pale and has a Glasgow Coma Scale score of 11/15. Her abdomen is generally tender, but there is no rigidity, rebound, or guarding. Bowel sounds are present and normal. Her respiratory rate is 36 breaths/minute, with no recession. Her heart rate is 160 bpm and her capillary refill time is 4 seconds. She is given a 20 mL/kg bolus of fluid. Blood tests show:

- haemoglobin 13 g/dL
- white cell count 22 × 10⁹/L
- C-reactive protein 25 mg/L
- sodium 120 mmol/L
- potassium 6.8 mmol/L
- urea 9.3 mmol/L
- creatinine 110 μmol/L.

Which is the single most important next investigation? ★

A Abdominal ultrasound scan

B Blood glucose

C CT scan of the head

D Serum ammonia

E Urine osmolality

22. A 3-year-old boy is in acute respiratory distress. There is no past history of note except that he has not been immunized. He has a temperature of 40°C, looks flushed and unwell, is drooling, and has an inspiratory stridor. His cough is muffled. A colleague asks for help examining the boy's throat. Which is the single most appropriate advice to give? ★

A Do not disturb the child, and call for senior help urgently

B Give nebulized budesonide and then examine the throat

C Go ahead and examine the throat, but have a laryngoscope and endotracheal tube to hand

D Go ahead and examine the throat straight away to help to make a diagnosis

E Site an intravenous line and give a dose of cefotaxime first, and then examine the throat

23. A 9-month-old boy has had a generalized seizure, which lasted for 5 minutes, during which he stared straight ahead and his arms and legs shook. He had been unwell for 12 hours with fever, runny nose, and cough. He has never had any fits before, and there is no family history of epilepsy. His development had been appropriate for his age, but in the last 6 weeks he has stopped pulling to stand or cruising round furniture. His temperature is 39°C and he has pharyngitis. A diagnosis of febrile convulsion is made. Which single feature in the history is least consistent with a diagnosis of febrile convulsion? ★

A The absence of previous febrile fits

B The age of the child

C The description of the seizure

D The developmental history

E The duration of the seizure

24. A 3-month-old baby girl has dry skin on her scalp, as shown in Plate 2.1 (see Colour Plate section). It has been present for the past 5 weeks and is getting progressively worse. Which is the single most likely diagnosis? ★

A Atopic eczema

B Impetigo

C Psoriasis

D Seborrhoeic dermatitis

E Tinea capitis

25. A 2.8 kg, 37-week-gestation baby girl has been treated briefly with phototherapy for jaundice. She is now 7 days old, breastfeeding well, and starting to regain weight. She has been off phototherapy for over 48 hours, and her bilirubin chart is shown in Plate 2.2 (see Colour Plate section). Her mother has heard someone mention that her baby has 'breast milk jaundice', and wants to know how she should continue to feed her baby. Which is the single most appropriate advice to give the mother? ★ ★

A She should continue to breastfeed, but also give some extra formula feeds to ensure a good milk intake to help to reduce the jaundice

B She should continue to breastfeed exclusively, as this is still the best milk for her baby, regardless of the jaundice, which is already improving

C She should give mainly formula milk for the next 3 weeks, with the occasional breastfeed to ensure an ongoing breast milk supply

D She should stop breastfeeding completely and change to a term formula to prevent the jaundice from worsening again

E She should stop breastfeeding for 48 hours to allow the jaundice level to fall further, and then restart

26. A 12-year-old girl has short stature. She had a birth weight of 2 kg at term and had a coarctation of the aorta repair in infancy. She has bilateral ptosis, a low posterior hairline, and multiple pigmented naevi. She is on the 0.4th centile for height and the 2nd centile for weight. Her mid-parental height is the 50th centile. Which single investigation is most likely to lead to a diagnosis? ★ ★

A Chest X-ray

B Coeliac screen

C Follicle-stimulating hormone and luteinizing hormone levels

D Karyotype

E MRI scan of brain

27. A 20-month-old South Asian boy has bow legs. He was breast-fed until the age of 6 months. The family live in a sixth-floor, two-bedroom flat, and his mother wears the hijab. He has mild genu varum bilaterally. His wrist X-ray is shown in Plate 2.3 (see Colour Plate section). Which single area of the X-ray shows the bony abnormalities that indicate the likely diagnosis? ★ ★

A Carpal bones

B Diaphyses of long bones

C Epiphyses of long bones

D Metacarpal bones

E Metaphyses of long bones

28. A 6-hour-old term baby boy weighs 2.54 kg. He has microcephaly, a flat occiput, upward-slanting palpebral fissures, a protruding tongue, a single palmar crease on the right hand but normal palmar creasing on the left, and a wide sandal gap. Which is the single most likely finding on neurological examination? ★ ★

A Absent Moro reflex

B Exaggerated Moro reflex

C Generalized hypertonia

D Generalized hypotonia

E Selective hypertonia of the lower limbs

29. A 7-year-old girl has had general malaise and pallor for the past 3 days. She is passing small amounts of urine infrequently. She was unwell the previous week with bloody diarrhoea, but this has now settled. Blood results show:

- haemoglobin 8.2 g/dL
- platelets 400 × 10^9/L
- white cell count 10.4 × 10^9/L
- sodium 135 mmol/L
- potassium 4.2 mmol/L
- urea 22 mmo/L
- creatinine 230 μmol/L
- C-reactive protein 11 mg/L.

Which single organism is the most likely cause of her illness? ★ ★

A *Clostridium difficile*

B *Escherichia coli*

C *Salmonella typhi*

D *Shigella sonnei*

E *Streptococcus pneumoniae*

30. An 8-year-old boy has had headaches for 12 months. They are usually left-sided and throbbing, and are made worse by noise and light. They last for around 12 hours, during which time he is nauseous but does not vomit. There are no obvious triggers. Treatment with paracetamol during attacks is of some benefit. He has one bad attack every 3 weeks on average, missing 1 to 2 days of school each time. Which is the single most appropriate next step in management? ★ ★

A Anti-emetic during attacks

B CT scan of the head

C Oral pizotifen

D Psychology referral

E Sumatriptan nasal spray

31. A 15-year-old boy is worried that he is shorter than all his friends and that he has not yet started puberty. He is otherwise well. His father started puberty at around the age of 14 years. The boy's parental heights are both on the 25th centile. His growth chart is shown in Plate 2.4 (see Colour Plate section). Which single aspect of his growth and pubertal development will be most likely to assist with diagnosis? ★ ★

A Axillary hair stage

B Height centile

C Height velocity centile

D Pubic hair stage

E Testicular size

32. A 5-year-old boy returned from visiting relatives in Bangladesh a week ago. He has had a temperature of 39°C, lower abdominal pain, and loose stool for 5 days. Blood tests show:

- haemoglobin 10.6 g/dL
- white cell count 17 x 10⁹/L
- lymphocyte count 13 x 10⁹/L
- platelet count 400 x 10⁹/L
- Gram-negative bacilli on blood culture.

Which is the single most likely diagnosis? ★ ★

A Dengue fever

B Leishmaniasis

C Leptospirosis

D Malaria

E Typhoid

33. A 4-month-old baby girl has had a temperature of 38°C for 2 days, and is consuming less than half of her usual amount during feeding. She has had an irritable cry and has been very unsettled for the last 24 hours. She has had three loose stools and two vomiting episodes in the last 12 hours. A lumbar puncture is performed which shows:

- clear colourless CSF
- glucose 2.9 mmol/L (blood glucose 5.4 mmol/L)
- protein 32 mg/dL
- white cell count 60/mm³ (90% mononuclear cells)
- red cell count 10/mm³
- Gram-negative staining

Intravenous access is established and she is started on IV ceftriaxone. Which is the single most appropriate medication to add? ★ ★

A Intravenous aciclovir

B Intravenous metronidazole

C Oral dexamethasone

D Oral isoniazid

E Oral rifampicin

34. A 25-week-gestation infant has just been delivered by spontaneous vaginal delivery. The full neonatal resuscitation team is present and the Resuscitaire® has been pre-warmed. The baby is handed to the team and they have started the clock. Which is the single most important action to take next? ★ ★ ★

A Assess the baby's initial Apgar score

B Dry the baby thoroughly and check the heart rate

C Intubate immediately and start ventilation breaths

D Put a hat on the baby's head and a plastic bag over his body

E Suction the mouth under direct vision using a laryngoscope

35. A 14-year-old girl has an osteosarcoma of her tibia. She has worsening pain in her leg. She is on regular oral paracetamol and ibuprofen. Which is the single most appropriate next treatment? ★ ★ ★

A Codeine phosphate

B Diazepam

C Diclofenac

D Hyoscine bromide

E Morphine sulphate

36. A newborn baby boy has a urethral meatus that emerges on the dorsum of the penis, as shown in Plate 2.5 (see Colour Plate section). He is able to pass a good stream of urine. Which single piece of advice should be given to his parents before discharge? ★ ★ ★

A He should not be circumcised

B He should not wear disposable nappies

C The foreskin should be retracted gently every day

D The penis should be cleaned with mild soapy water daily

E This is entirely normal and no further measures are needed

37. A 4-year-old boy was accidentally given IV cefuroxime 30 minutes ago, which was prescribed on the wrong drug chart. He has no relevant allergies and does not seem to have suffered any ill effects. The antibiotic has been crossed off his chart. His parents have now returned to the ward after being at home. Which is the single most appropriate course of action? ★ ★ ★

A Discuss the error at handover later in the day and write a reflective portfolio entry

B Do nothing further until the error has been discussed with a medical defence organization

C Explain the error and apologize to the parents and notify a senior colleague promptly

D Notify a senior colleague with a view to explaining the error to the parents later in the day

E Shred the incorrect prescription chart and write a new one before anyone else sees it

38. A 4-month-old girl has been irritable, with a temperature of 38°C for 2 days. She is diagnosed with a coliform urinary tract infection (UTI). Blood and cerebrospinal fluid cultures are negative. She responds to oral anibiotics and is afebrile after 24 hours. Which single set of investigations should be performed? ★ ★ ★

	Ultrasound of kidneys, ureters, and bladder	Dimercaptosuccinic acid (DMSA) renal isotope scan	Micturating cystourethrogram
A	No	No	No
B	Yes	No	No
C	Yes	Yes	No
D	Yes	No	Yes
E	Yes	Yes	Yes

39. A 14-year-old South Asian girl has had polyuria and polydipsia for 4 months. She has a body mass index of 28 kg/m² and dark, velvety pigmentation of the skin in her axillae. She has a random serum glucose concentration of 12 mmol/L and no blood ketones. Which is the single most likely diagnosis? ★ ★ ★

A Cushing's syndrome

B Diabetes insipidus

C Simple obesity

D Type 1 diabetes mellitus

E Type 2 diabetes mellitus

40. A 30-week-gestation infant is now 12 hours old. She was in good condition at birth and did not require resuscitation, although she did have some mild subcostal recession and needed 25% incubator oxygen. Over the past few hours she has developed increasing respiratory distress, with grunting, intercostal and subcostal recession, and an increasing oxygen requirement to 45%. Her blood gas analysis shows a respiratory acidosis, and her chest X-ray has a homogeneous ground-glass appearance with air bronchograms. She has just been intubated. Which is the single most appropriate medication to give immediately? ★ ★ ★

A Amoxicillin IV

B Dexamethasone IV

C Gentamicin IV

D Morphine infusion IV

E Surfactant via an endotracheal tube

41. A 6-year-old boy is 'always on the go' and finds it difficult to take turns. He is easily distracted and finds it difficult to focus on any task. His father says that he has no sense of danger and often runs across the main road without any care. He has difficulty following a series of simple instructions and is 1 year behind his peers in his numeracy and literacy skills. Which is the single most likely diagnosis? ★ ★ ★

A Attention deficit hyperactivity disorder (ADHD)

B Autism

C Dyspraxia

D Global developmental delay

E Oppositional defiant disorder

42. A 38-week-gestation, 3.1 kg baby is delivered by spontaneous vaginal delivery. The pregnancy has been complicated by poly-hydramnios. At birth, there are copious oral secretions and respiratory distress. The baby requires intubation and ventilation for respiratory distress, and continues to drool. It is not possible to pass a nasogastric tube to the estimated length required, and no acid reaction is obtained. Chest X-ray shows the nasogastric tube coiled in the oesophagus, a moderately large stomach bubble, and a normal gas pattern in the bowel. Which is the single most likely diagnosis? ★ ★ ★ ★

A H-type tracheo-oesophageal fistula

B Isolated oesophageal atresia

C Oesophageal atresia and tracheo-oesophageal fistula

D Oesophageal stenosis

E Oesophageal stricture

43. An 8-year-old boy had a throat infection and was given penicillin 2 days ago. He now has a red rash, which is peeling, on his trunk, sore red eyes, and has developed lesions on his mouth, shown in Plate 2.6 (see Colour Plate section). He looks unwell, and has a temperature of 39°C and a heart rate of 175 bpm. Which is the single most likely diagnosis? ★ ★ ★ ★

A Bullous impetigo

B Chickenpox

C Hand, foot, and mouth disease

D Measles

E Stevens–Johnson syndrome

44. A 9-week-old girl has had brief seizures for the last day, during which she stares straight ahead, her body shakes for a few seconds, and her right hand twitches. Pregnancy was normal but delivery was difficult due to shoulder dystocia. Her Apgar scores were 7 at 1 minute and 9 at 5 minutes. She has some pale areas of skin over her right thigh. She is afebrile. Urea and electrolytes, calcium, magnesium, and glucose are all normal. Lumbar puncture is bloodstained, with a protein concentration of 0.97 g/L (normal range is up to 0.4 g/L). Her EEG is normal. Her MRI brain scan is shown in Plate 2.7 (see Colour Plate section). Which is the single most likely diagnosis? ★ ★ ★ ★

A Benign neonatal seizures

B Hypoxic–ischaemic birth injury

C Infantile spasms

D Subdural haematoma

E Tuberous sclerosis

45. Five boys attend the same nursery. They are all aged 2 years 0 months and, by chance, they all have the same weight, of 12.5 kg (50th centile). Their parents compare their birth weights and gestations, which are listed as A–E below. Which single child is most at risk of later obesity? ★ ★ ★ ★

	Birth weight (centile)	Gestation (weeks)
A	1.5 kg (< 0.4th)	40
B	1.5 kg (50th)	30
C	2.0 kg (98th)	30
D	3.5 kg (50th)	40
E	5.0 kg (99.6th)	40

46. A 48-hour-old, 2.8 kg term baby girl has pallor, poor perfusion, cyanosis, and respiratory distress. She was born in good condition and was well for the first few hours of life. She has been intubated and ventilated, but her oxygen saturations remain in the range 70–80%, despite 100% oxygen and good chest movement. Her femoral pulses are not palpable. Which is the single most appropriate medication to commence next? ★ ★ ★ ★

A Dobutamine

B Dopamine

C Indomethacin

D Prostaglandin E$_2$

E Surfactant

47. A 4-year-old boy has had generalized oedema for 2 days and has 3+ proteinuria on dipstick testing of his urine. His blood pressure is 73/36 mmHg. His plasma albumin level is 18 g/L. All other blood tests, including his urea and electrolytes, are normal. He is started on high-dose daily oral prednisolone. Which single likelihood is there that he will respond to the treatment and not have any further relapses? ★ ★ ★ ★

A 3%

B 30%

C 50%

D 70%

E 90%

Extended Matching Questions

Causes of post-natal ward problems

For each baby with the clinical sign found on the baby check at approximately 36 hours old, choose the *single* most likely diagnosis from the list of options below. Each option may be used once, more than once, or not at all. ★

A Benign pustular melanosis

B Candidiasis

C Congenital melanocytic naevus

D Cutis marmorata

E Epstein

F Erythema toxicum neonatorum

G Milia

H Mongolian blue spot

I Neonatal herpes simplex virus

J Port-wine stain

K Stork mark

L Strawberry naevus

1. A 3.2 kg term baby has a raised, non-tender, well-demarcated, bright red lesion 0.5 cm in diameter on his right cheek.

2. A 2.9 kg 37-week-gestation baby has four small white cystic-looking nodules, 1–3 mm in diameter, along the midline of the palate.

3. A 4.2 kg 41-week-gestation baby has a widespread maculopapular rash with cream papules 1–3 mm in diameter on an erythematous macular base. The mother reports that the spots seem to 'come and go.'

4. A 3.6 kg 39-week-gestation baby has a macular, pink patch over the centre of the neck, forming a roughly triangular shape spreading out slightly towards the hairline.

5. A 3.4 kg South Asian baby has a large, blue-black macular discolouration approximately 5 cm in diameter over the base of the spine.

Causes of abdominal pain

For each child with abdominal pain, choose the *single* most likely diagnosis from the list of options below. Each option may be used once, more than once, or not at all. ★

A Coeliac disease

B Constipation

C Crohn's disease

D Gastroenteritis

E Henoch–Schönlein purpura

F Intussusception

G Lactose intolerance

H Mesenteric adenitis

I Migraine

J Non-organic recurrent abdominal pain

K Pneumonia

L Pyelonephritis

6. A 4-year-old boy has had central abdominal pain for 2 days. He has a palpable purpuric rash on his buttocks, and his ankles are swollen.

7. An 8-year-old girl has had lethargy, poor appetite, some weight loss, and right-sided abdominal pain for 5 months. Her stools tend to be loose. Her serum C-reactive protein concentration is 50 mg/L.

8. A 15-month-old boy has had sudden bouts of abdominal pain for 12 hours, when he screams inconsolably, draws his legs up, and becomes very pale. He has passed some reddish, jelly-like stool.

9. An 8-year-old girl has had intermittent, central abdominal pain on and off for 2 years. It lasts for a few minutes, during which she is pale. She has a normal bowel habit. She is growing along the 50th centile.

10. A 3-year-old girl has had poor growth since she was 9 months of age. Her weight and height are just below the 0.4th centile. She has recurrent abdominal pain and her stools are loose, pale, and difficult to flush. She has a distended abdomen.

Causes of cough

For each child with a cough, choose the *single* most likely diagnosis from the list of options below. Each option may be used once, more than once, or not at all. ★

A Anaphylaxis

B Bacterial tracheitis

C Cystic fibrosis

D Croup

E Epiglottitis

F Foreign body inhalation

G Gastro-oesophageal reflux disease

H Laryngomalacia

I Pertussis

J Tracheo-oesophageal fistula

11. A 14-month-old girl has had a cold for 2 days. She has a hoarse, barking cough and stridor at rest. Her temperature is 37.5°C and she has moderate respiratory distress.

12. A 3-month-old boy has had a cold and worsening cough for 1 week. When he coughs, he goes blue in the face. He has sub-conjunctival haemorrhages. His blood tests show a white cell count of 26×10^9/L, with a neutrophil count of 5.5×10^9/L and lymphocyte count of 19×10^9/L.

13. A 4-year-old boy is on stage 4 of the British Thoracic Society guidelines for asthma. He is compliant with his medication. He is asymptomatic during the day, but has significant nocturnal cough and wheeze. In the mornings he has 'really bad breath' and a hoarse voice. There is no family history of atopy. Immunoglobulin E (IgE) levels are normal, and tests for house dust mite and other common household allergens are negative.

14. A 1-day-old girl has large amounts of frothy mucus coming from her mouth and nose. During her first feed, she started to cough and went blue in the face. There was polyhydramnios during the pregnancy.

15. An 18-month-old boy suddenly starts coughing and goes blue in the face, with severe respiratory distress. He has moderate stridor and unilateral wheeze over the left lung, with normal air entry over the right lung.

Causes of floppiness in infants

For each of the following floppy infants, choose the *single* most likely diagnosis from the list below. Each option may be used once, more than once, or not at all. ★

A Congenital myotonic dystrophy

B Central nervous system malformation

C Down's syndrome

D Drug related

E Hypoglycaemia

F Hypothyroidism

G Hypoxic–ischaemic encephalopathy

H Inborn error of metabolism

I Myasthenia gravis

J Prader–Willi syndrome

K Prematurity

L Sepsis

M Spinal muscular atrophy

16. A 2-day-old boy born at 37 weeks' gestation has become jaundiced and floppy and has gone off his feeds in the last 6 hours. He was breastfeeding well until this point in time. His mother's membranes ruptured 36 hours before delivery.

17. A 2-day-old boy born at 38 weeks' gestation has been floppy and feeding poorly since birth. He has a harsh systolic cardiac murmur, which is loudest at the left sternal edge. He has tiny white speckles on his irises.

18. A 2-day-old boy born at 37 weeks' gestation has had surgery for exomphalos. He has macroglossia and earlobe creases. He is bottle-feeding and has become floppy and pale over the past hour.

19. A 2-day-old girl has been floppy since birth and has just had a 2-second generalized convulsion. She was born by emergency Caesarean section for acute placental abruption. Her Apgar scores were 1 at 1 minute, 3 at 5 minutes, and 4 at 10 minutes.

20. A 2-day-old South Asian boy born at 37 weeks' gestation has been floppy since he was 12 hours of age. His parents are consanguineous. His capillary blood glucose concentration is 3.2 mmol/L and his capillary pH is 7.1.

Causes of diarrhoea

For each patient with diarrhoea, choose the *single* most likely diagnosis from the list of options below. Each option may be used once, more than once, or not at all. ★

A Coeliac disease

B Cow's milk protein allergy

C Cystic fibrosis

D Galactosaemia

E Infectious enteritis

F Inflammatory bowel disease

G Intussusception

H Poor intake

I Sepsis

J Temporary lactose intolerance

21. A 7-day-old breastfed baby has lost 10% of her birth weight. She is lethargic and has a heart rate of 180 bpm and a capillary refill time of 4 seconds. Her temperature is 35°C. She has loose, watery stools. Her capillary blood glucose level is 3.6 mmol/L, serum sodium is 132 mmol/L, potassium is 5 mmol/L, urea is 8 mmol/L, creatinine is 70 µmol/L, bicarbonate is 13 mmol/L, and C-reactive protein is 60 mg/L.

22. A 6-year-old boy has had abdominal pain and bloody diarrhoea for 6 months. He has dropped 2 centiles in weight. His abdomen is generally tender. His full blood count shows a haemoglobin concentration of 8.2 g/dL, a mean corpuscular volume of 79 fL, a white cell count of 18×10^9/L, and a platelet count of 500×10^9/L.

23. A 6-month-old girl has vomiting, bloody diarrhoea, and abdominal distension, together with widespread eczema. She recently changed from breast milk to formula feeds.

24. A 10-year-old boy with type 1 diabetes has recurrent abdominal pain, oily loose stools, and recurrent episodes of hypoglycaemia.

25. A 3-month-old boy has had severe gastroenteritis, for which he has required intravenous rehydration. On reintroduction of feeds, his diarrhoea has worsened and he has increasing abdominal discomfort and distension and borborygmi.

Causes of limping in children

For each child with difficulty walking, choose the *single* most likely diagnosis from the list of options below. Each option may be used once, more than once, or not at all. ★

A Cerebral palsy

B Developmental dysplasia of the hip

C Henoch–Schönlein purpura

D Idiopathic thrombocytopaenic purpura

E Leukaemia

F Muscular dystrophy

G Myotonic dystrophy

H Perthes' disease

I Slipped upper femoral epiphyses

J Wilson's disease

26. A 3-year-old boy sat independently at 8 months, stood at 16 months, and now has frequent falls and has difficulty climbing stairs. He cannot jump when asked. He walks with short steps and sways his body from side to side.

27. A 2-year-old girl was born at 25 weeks' gestation. She sat at 12 months and stood at 18 months. She has increased tone and reflexes in her legs compared with her arms. When she walks, she is on tiptoe and adducts her legs. Both of her upper limbs flex when she walks.

28. A 6-year-old boy has had right-sided hip, groin, and intermittent knee pain for a week. He has limited internal rotation and abduction at the hip, and walks with a limp. There is no history of trauma and no recent illness. He is otherwise well. A full blood count and inflammatory markers are normal.

29. A 14-year-old boy is unsteady on his feet. He has become increasingly aggressive and has slurred speech. He has hepatosplenomegaly, a tremor at rest, and slowed movements.

30. A 4-year-old boy has been limping for 2 days. He has swelling over his left knee joint. He has a palpable purpuric rash on his buttocks. He had a cold a month ago.

Causes of decreased consciousness

For each child with a decreased conscious level, choose the *single* most likely diagnosis from the list of options below. Each option may be used once, more than once, or not at all. ★

A Cerebral oedema

B Encephalitis

C Metabolic defect

D Hypoxia

E Meningitis

F Migraine

G Non-convulsive status epilepticus

H Poisoning

I Stroke

J Wilson's disease

31. A 12-year-old boy has been generally unwell and has had a temperature for 10 days. Over the last 5 days he has developed a widespread, pruritic rash with erythematous papules, vesicles, and pustules, and some lesions are beginning to crust over. He is drowsy and confused, and he flexes to pain. There is no focal neurology. His capillary blood glucose concentration is 6 mmol/L.

32. A 6-month-old girl has had vomiting and diarrhoea for 1 day. She is drowsy and does not respond to voice, but flexes and moans when a cannula is inserted. She is moderately dehydrated. She has a capillary blood glucose concentration of 1.6 mmol/L and no ketones in her urine.

33. A 4-year-old girl with type 1 diabetes has diabetic ketoacidosis. She is treated for cardiovascular shock and started on an insulin infusion. Six hours later, she becomes unresponsive, bradycardic, and hypertensive.

34. A 4-year-old boy with sickle cell disease has fluctuating consciousness. He has a headache and also weakness of his right arm and leg.

35. A term baby is born by emergency Caesarean section after failure to progress in labour. The cardiotocograph (CTG) showed decreased variability and late decelerations for 2 hours prior to delivery. At birth, the baby is floppy, intermittently arches and extends his body, and does not suck.

Causes of discoloured urine

For each child presenting with red urine, choose the *single* most likely diagnosis from the list of options below. Each option may be used once, more than once, or not at all. ★ ★

A Alport's syndrome

B Coagulopathy

C Drug side-effect

D Fictitious

E Haemoglobinuria

F Henoch–Schönlein purpura

G Post-infectious glomerulonephritis

H Stones in urinary tract

I Thin basement membrane

J Trauma

K Tumour in urinary tract

L Urate crystals

M Urinary tract infection

36. A 4-month-old baby has had some orange-red stains in his wet nappy over the past 24 hours. His parents have never noticed this before. He has had a runny nose for the past 3 weeks, but is otherwise well and thriving. He is breastfed. Examination is normal. Urine dipstick is negative for glucose, blood, protein, ketones, leucocytes, and nitrites.

37. A 4-year-old boy has had dark urine for 3 days. He is otherwise well. He was unwell 2 weeks ago with a cough, cold, and sore throat, and had a course of amoxicillin. Examination is normal, except for several mobile upper cervical lymph nodes. His blood pressure is 110/53 mmHg. A urine dipstick shows 2+ blood and 1+ protein.

38. A 10-month-old baby has a fever of 39°C and is irritable. He has had two previous episodes of fever when there was no obvious cause, but no tests were done. He appears miserable and has several mobile upper cervical lymph nodes. A urine dipstick shows 2+ blood, 1+ protein, 3+ leucocytes, and 2+ nitrites.

39. A 5-year-old girl has had red urine for 24 hours. Both of her parents have had colds recently, and her 2-year-old brother was admitted to hospital 2 days ago with suspected meningitis, for which the whole family have been given an antibiotic. A urine dipstick is negative.

40. A 10-year-old boy has been followed up in the paediatric outpatient department because dipsticks of his urine have been persistently positive for blood (usually 1+), but otherwise negative. The first dipstick was done 1 year ago when he had enuresis. Urine culture was negative and microscopy showed red cells but no casts. All further blood tests and a renal ultrasound have been normal. His enuresis has now resolved and he is otherwise well. He has never had any visible abnormality of the urine. His blood pressure is 110/62 mmHg. Two family members have had long-standing isolated haematuria. There is no family history of deafness.

Causes of fits, faints, and funny turns

For each child presenting with a paroxysmal episode, choose the *single* most likely diagnosis from the list of options below. Each option may be used once, more than once, or not at all. ★ ★ ★

A Benign childhood epilepsy with centro-temporal spikes (rolandic)

B Breath-holding attack

C Childhood absence epilepsy

D Juvenile myoclonic epilepsy

E Night terrors

F Pseudo-seizure

G Self-gratification phenomenon

H Syncope

I Temporal lobe epilepsy

J West syndrome (infantile spasms)

41. A 10-month-old boy is having episodes during which he suddenly jerks his head forwards and extends his arms upwards. He was sitting on his own 2 months ago, but now needs support to sit. His babbling has reduced. His EEG has a chaotic appearance.

42. A 15-month-old girl has had 10 episodes over the past 2 months when she suddenly became silent, usually after a cry, and then became unconscious for a few seconds. On two occasions there were brief clonic limb movements towards the end of the episode. She rapidly returned to normal. All of the episodes were triggered by frustration or pain. She has always been afebrile.

43. A 3-year-old girl has recurrent episodes at nursery lasting for 5 to 10 minutes during story time, when she becomes red and sweaty and her eyes glaze over. She is usually sitting on the mat with her legs outstretched and her body rocks backwards and forwards. When picked up, she immediately returns to normal.

44. A 9-year-old boy has had three episodes that occur on waking. He first feels a tingling on one side of the mouth, and then makes a gurgling noise and cannot speak properly. He finally makes small jerking movements, which spread from his arm to his leg on the left side. Afterwards he is sleepy for several hours.

45. A 12-year-old girl 'goes blank' for several seconds at a time 20 or 30 times in the school day. Afterwards she has lost the thread of any conversation or class discussion. She tends to make small, repetitive hand movements during these episodes.

ANSWERS

Single Best Answers

1. E ★   OHCS 9th edn → p. 136

Heart murmurs are heard in many neonates. It is important to know the characteristics that signify congenital heart disease. Significant murmurs are usually harsh sounding and may be associated with thrills. In this case, the systolic murmur indicates a lesion where turbulent flow occurs in systole (i.e. aortic stenosis, pulmonary stenosis, ventricular septal defect, and atrial septal defect). The thrill at the left sternal edge indicates turbulent flow in the area of the septum. A patent ductus has a continuous murmur as blood flows across the ductus in both systole and diastole. Normal femoral pulses argue against a severe aortic stenosis or coarctation.

For an excellent learning resource on congenital heart disease that explains the anatomy by likening it to the rooms of a house, see the Children's Heart Institute website:

→ http://childrensheartinstitute.org/educate/eduhome.htm

2. E ★   OHCS 9th edn → p. 151

The mild upper respiratory symptoms are not a reason for delaying immunization. The red area and irritability after the previous immunization are normal, and the mother should have been counselled to expect this.

→ www.dh.gov.uk/en/Publicationsandstatistics/Publications/
PublicationsPolicyAndGuidance/DH_079917 ('*The Green Book*'; see Chapter 6. This is a key UK resource for immunization).

3. E ★   OHCS 9th edn → pp. 188–189

This child has diabetic ketoacidosis (DKA). Fluid management has been appropriate so far, but now that she has passed urine, potassium needs to be added to her maintenance fluid, otherwise she will rapidly become hypokalaemic. Her glucose level is falling at a rate of 2.5 mmol/hour, which is about right. It should not be allowed to fall faster than 5 mmol/hour. Once her blood glucose concentration reaches 14–17 mmol/L, you would change her IV fluid to one containing dextrose and potassium. The slight fall in her calcium level is not significant. The British Society for Paediatric Endocrinology and Diabetes has published guidelines on the management of DKA in children:

→ www.bsped.org.uk/clinical/docs/DKAGuideline.pdf

4. C ★

A common mistake in the management of constipation is to discontinue the laxative too quickly. It should have been continued for about 6 months to allow time for the distended 'baggy' colon to return to normal, and this needs to be explained to the parents at the outset. This girl's constipation has relapsed, and her soiling is due to overflow. The use of suppositories in young children should be avoided if at all possible. Movicol® is an osmotic laxative (containing ethylene glycol particles).

→ http://adc.bmj.com/cgi/content/full/94/2/156 →http://guidance.nice.org.uk/CG99/NICEGuidance/pdf/English

5. B ★   OHCS 9th edn → p. 211

This is primary monosymptomatic nocturnal enuresis, and the boy should do well with an enuresis alarm. He should be followed up every few weeks while using it. He has not made progress after keeping a star chart for 4 weeks, so it is best not to persist with this on its own, but it could be combined with alarm treatment. Desmopressin could be used in the short term if he is not dry by the time of the cub camp. Imipramine is a second-line drug treatment because of the higher incidence of side-effects. Oxybutynin would only be appropriate if there were symptoms of detrusor instability (e.g. daytime urgency and frequency). Enuresis is common.

→ http://guidance.nice.org.uk/CG111/NICEGuidance/pdf/English

6. C ★   OHCS 9th edn → p. 234

This child is moderately dehydrated due to gastroenteritis. According to the NICE traffic light system, he should have an initial trial of oral rehydration therapy (ORT), especially as he is not vomiting. The aim should be for him to drink 50 mL/kg over 4 hours. If he is not managing to drink this amount, change to nasogastric ORT. If he is vomiting, use IV fluid. If he was severely dehydrated, you would initially give 20 mL/kg IV 0.9% saline.

→ http://www.nice.org.uk/CG84

7. B ★   OHCS 9th edn → p. 136

Up to 60% of newborn infants have audible but benign heart murmurs in the first 24 hours of life. These are due to the increase in pulmonary blood flow that occurs after birth in association with relatively high pulmonary vascular resistance. As the pulmonary vascular resistance drops, the murmur disappears.

8. D ★   OHCS 9th edn → p. 166

This child has signs of a flitting polyarthritis—that is, arthritis affecting more than four joints that comes and goes. She also has the rash of erythema marginatum. Coupled with the recent history of a sore throat, this fits the criteria for rheumatic fever. Either two major criteria (which both of these fit) or one major and two minor criteria (fever is a minor criterion) are needed. Rheumatic fever is now less common in the UK, possibly due to the use of antibiotics to treat streptococcal throat infections. However, it is still seen in other parts of the world. It is caused by a cross-sensitivity reaction to Group A streptococcus in susceptible individuals.

9. A ★ OHCS 9th edn → p. 170

Appendicitis is the commonest cause of acute abdomen, and should not be forgotten in children. It is rare in children under 5 years, and becomes more common with increasing age thereafter. The classic presentation is with central, colicky abdominal pain, which then spreads to the right iliac fossa and becomes constant in nature. However, the pain may not always be in a classic position, so other clues need to be looked for. Vomiting is almost universal, together with associated anorexia. Loose stool and dysuria may occur as a result of irritation from the inflamed appendix, so in a child with other symptoms one should not automatically assume that these are due to simple gastroenteritis or urinary tract infection.

10. B ★ OHCS 9th edn → p. 684

Barlow's test and Ortolani's test are used to check for developmental dysplasia of the hip. Barlow's test should be performed first (Barlow's = Back). Hold the thigh in one hand while stabilizing the pelvis with the other. With the leg in the midline, push back gently. If the hip is dislocat-*able*, the femoral head will pop out of the acetabulum. Then perform Ortolani's test (Ortolani's = Out). Holding the leg in the same way, gently and steadily abduct the leg as far as you can, pushing up gently with your fingers on the greater trochanter. If the hip is dislocat*ed*, you will feel the femoral head pop back into the acetabulum, or the hip will simply not abduct fully.

11. D ★ OHCS 9th edn → pp. 218–219

It is important to know some of the common developmental milestones for children aged 0–5 years in all four developmental areas. In this case development is normal apart from the lack of language.

→ www.gpnotebook.co.uk/simplepage.cfm?ID=1946550277

12. C ★

As the law stands, children under the age of 16 years can consent to treatment if they are judged to be Gillick competent, but they cannot refuse treatment. A person with parental responsibility gives consent on behalf of a child under 16 years of age. As the mother is the only person with parental responsibility, it is she who should decide future treatment. However, in practice every effort is made to help all of the parties to reach a decision together.

→ www.gmc-uk.org/guidance/ethical_guidance/children_guidance/index.asp

13. **A** ★   OHCS 9th edn → p. 136

These are symptoms of heart failure—shortness of breath and sweating, which is worse on effort (e.g. during feeding), tachypnoea, tachycardia, and hepatomegaly. This baby is also showing signs of shock. Heart failure often presents in neonates at about 4–6 weeks of age, when the pulmonary vascular resistance falls.

14. **B** ★

Babies can lose up to 10% of their birth weight in the first week, but should have regained their birth weight by 2 weeks of age. This baby has lost 150 g, which is 5.5% of 2.7 kg. Although breastfeeding was slow initially, it is now going well and should be encouraged.

15. **A** ★   OHCS 9th edn → p. 166

Children who have congenital heart lesions are at risk of infective endocarditis. Poor dental hygiene is a risk factor.

16. **D** ★

These features point to a diagnosis of rickets. This is especially common in African-Caribbean and South Asian children in the UK who are breast-fed for a prolonged period. This is because dark-skinned people absorb less sunlight and there is less conversion of 7-dehydrocholesterol to pre-vitamin D_3. This results in even lower levels of vitamin D in breast milk.

→ www.patient.co.uk/health/Vitamin-D-Deficiency.htm

17. **C** ★   OHCS 9th edn → p. 146

The concern here is the possibility of non-accidental injury. When thinking about the mechanism of an injury, it is vital always to take into account the child's developmental stage. In this case, consider whether a 7-month-old child is capable of climbing out of a cot.

18. **E** ★   OHCS 9th edn → p. 162

It is important always to reconsider a diagnosis of 'asthma' in children who do not respond to treatment, and to consider referral for special-ist opinion. In this case, the recurrent infections, nasal discharge, poor growth, and clubbing suggest cystic fibrosis. A sweat test is diagnostic for this and should be done. Lung function and a CT scan of the chest may be performed following diagnosis in order to obtain additional information, but the important step is making the diagnosis.

→ www.patient.co.uk/doctor/Cystic-Fibrosis.htm

19. B ★   OHCS 9th edn → pp. 178–179

Nephrotic syndrome is a triad of hypoalbuminaemia, proteinuria, and oedema. It often presents with periorbital oedema just after a viral infection, and it is important to dip a urine sample to look for the proteinuria, otherwise it may be dismissed as an allergic reaction, of which angioedema may be a variety. The lack of blood in the urine rules out glomerulonephritis, and systemic lupus erythematosus (SLE) is rare. The presence of oedema rules out benign postural proteinuria.

20. E ★

Tension pneumothorax must always be considered in acutely ill asthmatic patients who deteriorate suddenly.

21. B ★   OHCS 9th edn → pp. 188–189

With any sick child, remember ABCDEFG—Airway, Breathing, Circulation and Don't Ever Forget Glucose. This girl is shocked and dehydrated, and has altered consciousness and a relative hyponatraemia and hyperkalaemia caused by hyperglycaemia. The diagnosis is diabetic ketoacidosis, and a capillary blood glucose test will confirm this.

22. A ★   OHCS 9th edn → p. 158

This child is very likely to have epiglottitis. He has not been immunized so is not protected against *Haemophilus influenzae* type B, and he shows signs of upper airway obstruction. Any disturbance may cause deterioration, and an attempt to examine the throat may cause fatal respiratory arrest. Intubation is difficult due to the swollen epiglottis, and occasionally emergency tracheostomy is required. Senior anaesthetic and ENT help should be summoned urgently.

23. D ★   OHCS 9th edn → p. 206

There seems to be developmental regression (at least for gross motor skills), which would not be consistent with a febrile convulsion. Other more serious diagnoses should be considered.

24. D ★   OHCS 9th edn → p. 596

This is a severe case of seborrhoeic dermatitis affecting the scalp (also known as 'cradle cap' in young children). Note the thick yellow scale and crust.

25. B ★★   OHCS 9th edn → p. 115

The benefits of breast milk far outweigh any disadvantages related to mild jaundice. Although it is not entirely clear why breastfed babies develop persistent jaundice, these babies rarely, if ever, have levels of unconjugated bilirubin high enough to cause kernicterus.

26. D ★★ OHCS 9th edn → p. 655

The clinical features, namely female gender, short stature, ptosis, and a left heart defect, point to Turner's syndrome. The latter is an XO karyotype, with only one X chromosome, and it is diagnosed by chromosome analysis. This should always be considered in girls with short stature.

27. E ★★

The wrist X-ray shows widened, frayed, and cupped metaphyses of the radius and ulna. These changes are typical of rickets, and are usually combined with osteopenia. The metaphysis is the growth plate, and it lies between the diaphysis (the shaft of the long bone) and the epiphysis (the end of the bone). This area fails to mineralize normally in the growing child, due to low vitamin D levels. The aetiology is most probably a combination of initial low vitamin D stores secondary to maternal deficiency, and ongoing low sunlight exposure.

→ www.bmj.com/content/340/bmj.b5664

28. D ★★ OHCS 9th edn → p. 152

These are the classic phenotypic features of a baby with trisomy 21 (Down's syndrome). The consistent neurological finding in babies with trisomy 21 is generalized hypotonia—they are floppy babies.

29. B ★★ OHCS 9th edn → p. 176

This is haemolytic uraemic syndrome, which is usually caused by verocytotoxin-producing E. coli. The toxin causes haemolysis and renal failure.

→ www.hpa.org.uk/web/HPAweb&Page&HPAwebAutoListName/Page/1296687744200

30. C ★★ OHCS 9th edn → p. 201

The headache is typical of migraine. The long history and lack of any suggestive features effectively rule out a space-occupying lesion. For this reason, and because there is a clear clinical diagnosis, a CT scan is not indicated. The frequency of bad attacks (more than once a month) interfering with school justifies prophylactic treatment, and pizotifen is probably most commonly used in the UK, and is licensed for this age group. However, it is not of proven benefit. This boy is too young to be treated with sumatriptan nasal spray (although sumatriptan can be given orally).

→ http://ihs-classification.org/en/02_klassifikation/02_teil1/01.00.00_migraine.html (International Headache Society)

Ryan S (2007). Medicines for migraine. *Arch Dis Child Educ Pract Ed* **92**: ep50–ep55.

31. E ★ ★ OHCS 9th edn → p. 180

This boy is most likely to have constitutional delay in growth and puberty. As testicular enlargement is the first sign of puberty in boys, measurement of testicular volume (using an orchidometer, consisting of a string of testicle-shaped beads of different volumes) will indicate whether he has started puberty even in the absence of other signs. If his testicular size is greater than 4mL, you can reassure him that he has entered puberty, and that the other signs and a growth spurt will follow. The pubertal growth spurt is a late event in boys. All of the other items are relevant and should be recorded.

32. E ★ ★ OHCS 9th edn → p. 168

All of these are tropical infections that can occur in South Asia and cause high fever. Typhoid is caused by *Salmonella enterica* serotype Typhi, a Gram-negative bacillus. It is transmitted from human to human through water or food contaminated with faeces. The incubation period is usually 7–14 days, and the first phase of the illness causes increasing fever, headache, malaise, anorexia, abdominal pain, and usually diarrhoea in children. Classic features of the disease, such as rose spots, generally do not appear until the second week. Diagnosis is based on finding the bacteria on blood culture. Dengue fever is a viral infection that is transmitted via mosquito bites. The incubation period is about 4–7 days, and infection causes an acute febrile illness with headache, myalgia, and joint pain. There is a risk of developing a haemorrhagic illness as the fever subsides. Leishmaniasis is a parasitic disease that is spread by the bite of infected sand flies. It can have a very long incubation period and abrupt or gradual onset of symptoms, which typically include fever, weight loss, and hepatosplenomegaly. Malaria is a common illness in travellers returning to the UK. It is a mosquito-borne parasitic infection caused by *Plasmodium* species. After an incubation period of 1 to 2 weeks, symptoms of fever, rigors, myalgia, headache, cough, and diarrhoea develop. Malaria is diagnosed by seeing the parasites on thick and thin blood films or by a rapid antigen test. Leptospirosis has a long incubation period of 2 to 3 weeks, and is typically contracted from water that has been contaminated with the urine of animals, such as rats. The acute phase is similar to that of typhoid. However, *Leptospira* species are spirochaete bacteria.

33. A ★ ★ OHCS 9th edn → pp. 201–202

This baby's presentation raises concern about the possibility of meningoencephalitis, and ceftriaxone is a broad-spectrum antibiotic that should be started if this is suspected. The cerebrospinal fluid (CSF) picture confirms this, with a raised white cell count. However, it indicates that a viral cause is likely, with a near normal glucose level, normal protein, and mostly mononuclear cells seen. Aciclovir is an antiviral medication that can be used to treat herpes simplex, which is the most likely cause of viral encephalitis in this age group. It should be started alongside broad-spectrum antibiotics whenever viral encephalitis is thought to be a possibility. Infection with anaerobes is very unlikely in an otherwise well child, so metronidazole will offer no benefit. Intravenous dexamethasone is used at the time of giving antibiotics in bacterial meningitis, to reduce the incidence of neurological complications. Isoniazid is used to treat TB. Rifampicin is sometimes used as chemoprophylaxis in cases of meningococcal meningitis.

34. D ★ ★ ★   OHCS 9th edn → p. 107

Pre-term babies lose heat very easily. Placing them immediately into a plastic bag has been shown to be most effective in conserving heat. Hypothermia is associated with a worse outcome and should be avoided.

→ www.resus.org.uk/pages/nls.pdf

35. A ★ ★ ★

Analgesia should not be forgotten in children who are in pain. There is well-published guidance on a step-wise approach to analgesia, starting with simple treatments and adding in further treatment. However, different analgesics are effective for different types of pain. Bony pain responds well to non-steroidal anti-inflammatory drugs (NSAIDs), and this girl is already on one of these, so another is not appropriate. In malignancy, opioids are often needed, and simple opioids such as codeine should be tried first. Diazepam and hyoscine may be adjunctive treatments in symptom control in palliative care, but are not analgesics.

→ www.who.int/cancer/palliative/painladder/en/index.html

36. A ★ ★ ★   OHCS 9th edn → p. 132

This shows epispadias, where the urethral meatus comes out on the dorsum of the penis. More common is hypospadias, where the urethral meatus comes out on the ventral aspect of the penis and is often narrowed. In reconstruction of both, the foreskin may be needed, so it is vital to warn the parents not to have the child circumcised until the surgeon has made an operative assessment. Otherwise there is no increased risk of infection, and it is always better not to retract the foreskin of babies.

37. C ★ ★ ★

Drug errors are one of the commonest types of error in paediatric practice. Anyone can make an error, and the best way to improve patient safety is to improve systems and training. The parents should receive an early explanation and apology. Any such incident is serious, and you should promptly involve a senior colleague. You may think that no harm has been done, but there may be wider issues to consider. Reflective portfolio entries and notification of your defence society are often appropriate, but are not the most important actions.

→ www.nrls.npsa.nhs.uk/resources/?entryid45=65077

38. B ★ ★ ★   OHCS 9th edn → p. 174

Note that recommendations for the investigation of UTIs in children have changed in England and Wales recently with the publication of the National Institute for Health and Clinical Excellence (NICE) guidelines. Investigation is now generally more conservative. This child is under 6 months of age, but her UTI was typical and not recurrent, and she responded to treatment within 48 hours. Therefore she needs a renal ultrasound scan, which should be performed within 6 weeks, to look for anatomical abnormalities, but she does not require any other imaging.

→ http://guidance.nice.org.uk/CG54

39. E ★ ★ ★   OHCS 9th edn → pp. 156, 186

The incidence of type 2 diabetes in children is rising, although it is still far less common than type 1 diabetes. The risk is increased in children who are overweight, who have a family history of type 2 diabetes, and who are of South Asian origin. The velvety skin in this girl's axillae is characteristic of acanthosis nigricans, a finding in insulin resistance and obesity.

40. E ★ ★ ★   OHCS 9th edn → p. 118

Surfactant treatment via an endotracheal tube is the most important treatment for respiratory distress syndrome, and should be given as rescue treatment as soon as the baby has been intubated. Antibiotics should also be commenced (if this has not already been done) after blood cultures have been taken, and morphine may be needed for sedation on the ventilator.

41. A ★ ★ ★   OHCS 9th edn → p. 212

ADHD is part of a spectrum of hyperactive behaviour. It is characterized by lack of concentration and by impulsivity, with or without hyperactivity, that pervades all areas of the child's life. It is more common in children with learning difficulties. Autism is also part of a spectrum, characterized by impaired social interaction, impaired imagination, and a limited repertoire of interests. Dyspraxia is a developmental coordination disorder. Oppositional defiant disorder is a pattern of defiant, disobedient, and hostile behaviour.

→ http://guidance.nice.org.uk/CG72

42. C ★ ★ ★ ★   OHCS 9th edn → p. 130

This is a typical picture of oesophageal atresia, with polyhydramnios, 'blowing bubbles', respiratory distress, and inability to pass a nasogastric tube. Approximately 92% of oesophageal atresias are also associated with a tracheo-oesophageal fistula. The H-type, in which both the oesophagus and the trachea are patent but there is a small connection between them, is rare and is often diagnosed later.

43. E ★★★★ OHCS 9th edn → p. 601

The combination of a sick child, an erythematous rash with exfoliation, and severe mucous membrane involvement indicates Stevens–Johnson syndrome. This is associated with some viral infections and certain drugs, including penicillins.

44. E ★★★★ OHCS 9th edn → p. 638

The MRI scan shows subependymal nodules in the left ventricle. This, combined with seizures and hypopigmented skin lesions, is strongly suggestive of tuberous sclerosis.

45. A ★★★★ OHCS 9th edn → p. 156

Catch-up growth for weight in early childhood is a risk factor for obesity.

→ www.pubmedcentral.nih.gov/articlerender.fcgi?tool=pubmed&pub medid=1645067

46. D ★★★★ OHCS 9th edn → p. 136

Prostaglandin E_2 should be commenced because the clinical presentation is consistent with a duct-dependent congenital cardiac lesion where the duct has just closed. This means that blood can no longer flow around the body. It should cause the duct to reopen until something definitive can be done. The duct typically closes at around 48 hours of age, so a duct-dependent lesion should always be considered in babies who collapse at this age.

47. B ★★★★ OHCS 9th edn → pp. 178–179

This boy almost certainly has minimal change nephrotic syndrome (MCNS), given his age, normal blood pressure, lack of haematuria, and normal renal function and other blood tests. Around 95% of children with MCNS will respond to steroids, although most relapse at some point. The long-term outlook is good.

Eddy AA and Symons JM (2003). Nephrotic syndrome in childhood. *Lancet* **362**: 629–639.

Extended Matching Questions

1. L ★

These are bright red and irregular. They enlarge in size initially and then shrink and disappear by the age of 4 to 5 years. They are distinguished from port-wine stains (capillary vascular naevus) by the fact that the latter are flat and a purplish colour, like port wine. Stork mark is the name for a capillary dilatation on the nape of the neck.

2. E ★

These are seen in over half of newborns and are caused by entrapment of fluid during development of the palate. They disappear within a few weeks and are harmless.

3. F ★

This is seen in about half of newborns and, despite the name, is completely harmless. Classically, there are small pustule-like spots on a red base and the fleeting nature is characteristic. The main differential is a staphylococcal skin infection, which has smaller, non-mobile spots.

4. K ★

5. H ★

This mark is common in dark-skinned babies, and is sometimes mistaken for bruising. The blue colour is caused by melanocytes in the skin, and it usually occurs over the lumbo-sacral area, although it can occur elsewhere.

General feedback on 1–5: OHCS 9th edn → p. 121

6. E ★

The characteristic distribution of the rash on the buttocks combined with swelling of the joints suggests Henoch–Schönlein purpura.

7. C ★

The chronic history, loose stools, and weight loss together with raised inflammatory markers suggest Crohn's disease.

8. F ★

This is a surgical emergency and it should be suspected in children aged 5–18 months, although it can occur at an older age. The intermittent painful episodes with pallor are classic, as is the 'redcurrant-jelly' stool, although this is a late sign.

9. J ★

The long history of normal growth is very reassuring and suggests a non-organic cause.

10. A ★

This causes poor growth with malabsorption stools that are loose and bulky. Classically, it causes abdominal distension and the child is miserable. It occurs after the introduction of gluten-containing foods, but can otherwise occur at any age.

General feedback on 5–10: OHCS 9th edn → pp. 170–171

11. D ★

Croup, or viral laryngotracheobronchitis, is common. It causes symptoms of a cold together with laryngeal oedema. This causes a harsh cough, typically with the sound of 'barking like a seal' and easy to recognize, and stridor.

12. I ★

Whooping cough has not disappeared completely, despite immunization programmes. It occurs in young children who have not yet been fully immunized, and it can be serious. The bouts of coughing are paroxysmal, severe, and prolonged, and may result in apnoea. The characteristic finding is a marked lymphocytosis on blood tests.

13. G ★

Although asthma is common, many children who are diagnosed with it in fact have other conditions. In this case, the normal investigations and lack of family history call the diagnosis into question. The bad breath and the fact that symptoms only occur at night when lying down are clues to reflux.

14. J ★

The mucus indicates that this baby cannot swallow secretions. The choking during her first feed also indicates that she is having problems swallowing. The term 'tracheo-oesophageal fistula' refers to a number of different patterns, but in the commonest types there is oesophageal atresia, causing inability to swallow. In this case there will be polyhydramnios in pregnancy because the fetus cannot swallow amniotic fluid.

15. F ★

During play, young children frequently inhale small objects, such as peanuts or small parts of toys. If this is witnessed, it is reasonably easy to make a diagnosis. Unilateral wheeze confirms the diagnosis, as there is selective obstruction of the airways on one side.

General feedback on 11–15: OHCS 9th edn → pp. 158–160, 164

16. L ★

Prolonged rupture of membranes is a risk factor for sepsis. Poor feeding and jaundice may be signs of sepsis, and this should always be considered in unwell newborns.

17. C ★

Babies with Down's syndrome are always floppy. Dysmorphic features may be subtle, such as the white flecks on the iris (Brushfield spots). Heart defects are also common in Down's syndrome.

18. E ★

This baby has Beckwith–Wiedemann syndrome, which is a rare overgrowth disorder. Babies with this syndrome are large for dates, have large organs, and may have exomphalos because of bowel overgrowth. A characteristic feature is earlobe creases. These babies become hypoglycaemic because of increased insulin levels, in the same way that babies of diabetic mothers do.

19. G ★

This describes the brain damage that occurs because of oxygen deprivation at birth. This is a risk in abruption, and the poor Apgar scores indicate that this baby's health suffered from the start.

20. H ★

Consanguinity (having a child with a close relative) increases the risk of inborn errors of metabolism, which tend to follow a pattern of autosomal recessive inheritance. They often cause hypoglycaemia and acidosis.

21. I ★

Sepsis is the main diagnosis to consider in unwell babies. Hypothermia can be seen rather than fever, in addition to a range of metabolic disturbances. This baby is shocked and unwell.

22. F ★

Bloody diarrhoea, weight loss, and anaemia all indicate a significant pathology. There are signs of inflammation on blood tests, with an elevated white cell count and platelet count.

23. B ★

The timing of the change from breast milk to formula feeds is important here.

24. A ★

Type 1 diabetes is an autoimmune condition and there is an increased risk of other immune-mediated diseases, such as coeliac disease, which is characterized by features of malabsorption.

25. J ★

Following gastroenteritis, the gut can take some time to heal completely, and there may be a transient lactose intolerance. This will cause symptoms of malabsorption.

General feedback on 21–25: OHCS 9th edn → pp. 168, 171

26. F ★

Duchenne's muscular dystrophy affects boys and usually presents at around 1–6 years of age with weakness and a waddling gait. These boys often have motor developmental delay and may be late in starting to walk.

27. A ★

Premature babies are at increased risk of spastic diplegia, a form of cerebral palsy that affects the lower limbs more than the upper limbs. There is delayed development and hypertonia, causing scissoring of the legs.

28. H ★

This is an osteochondritis of the femoral head. It is seen mainly in 4- to 7-year-olds, and occurs in boys more often than in girls. It causes a painful limp with limited hip movement. The normal blood tests rule out leukaemia or idiopathic thrombocytopaenic purpura. Slipped upper femoral epiphysis is painless and occurs in older children.

29. J ★

This is a rare disease, and it causes neurological and liver abnormalities, which may not be seen at the same time. It occurs in older children.

30. C ★

The classic presentation of Henoch–Schönlein purpura is a purpuric rash on the lower limbs and buttocks of a well child, who also has joint pain and swelling. It typically occurs a few weeks after a viral illness, although the cause is unknown.

General feedback on 26–30: OHCS 9th edn → pp. 214, 642, 682

31. B ★

The rash appears to be viral in nature here, and is likely to be caused by herpes simplex virus, which can lead to the development of encephalitis.

32. C ★

Inborn errors of metabolism can present in many ways, but should be considered in infants who present with decreased consciousness. The clues here are hypoglycaemia in the absence of ketones, which mean that the body needs fuel but cannot mount the normal metabolic pathways and produce ketones.

33. A ★

Cerebral oedema is a recognized risk in diabetic ketoacidosis if too much fluid is given too rapidly. It is important to treat shock, but fluid management needs to be meticulous.

34. I ★

Sickle cell disease causes blockage of the small blood vessels as the sickled cells cannot flow smoothly. In the brain, this can lead to areas of ischaemia and stroke.

35. D ★

An abnormal CTG is an indication of hypoxia *in utero*.

General feedback on 31–35: OHCS 9th edn → pp. 183, 189, 202

36. L ★★

Urate crystals can sometimes resemble blood stains on the nappy, but usually have an orange-red quality that is quite characteristic. If there is any doubt, the red area can be eluted into some water in a specimen pot and tested with a urine dipstick, which will indicate the presence of any blood. The test will be negative if urate crystals are the cause.

37. G ★★

This is typical of post-streptococcal glomerulonephritis. Note that the antistreptolysin O titre is raised. The urine is typically described as 'smoky' or 'like Coca Cola.'

38. M ★★

The urine dipstick test strongly suggests a UTI. The two previous febrile episodes may also have been UTIs. Other causes of fever should be considered in a young child who is irritable with a high fever, including septicaemia and meningitis (depending on how ill the child appears).

39. C ★★

This child is being treated with rifampicin as meningococcal prophylaxis. This drug can turn the urine pink, and the parents should have been warned about this.

40. I ★★

Isolated persistent haematuria with minimal or no proteinuria, normal renal function, and a family history of similar benign problems suggests thin basement membrane disease, otherwise known as benign familial haematuria. It is important to make sure that there is no family history of deafness (which suggests Alport's syndrome) or renal failure (which might indicate a more serious cause).

General feedback on 36–40: OHCS 9th edn → pp. 174, 178

41. J ★★★

West syndrome is otherwise known as infantile spasms, so the age is a pointer. The flexor spasms, developmental regression, and characteristic EEG appearance (hypsarrhythmia) all point to the diagnosis.

42. B ★★★

The fact that all of the episodes were triggered by frustration or pain makes epilepsy very unlikely, and strongly suggests breath-holding. The age and description are typical. Brief clonic movements may occur.

43. G ★★★

This is a form of masturbation. The age and description are typical, as is the fact that the girl returns to normal when self-stimulation is prevented.

44. A ★★★

Nocturnal seizures that progress from the arm to the leg on one side are typical of this condition.

45. C ★★★

Absences are described, and the small movements (which can also occur around the face or lips) are a helpful clue, although they are not always present.

General feedback on 40–45: OHCS 9th edn → pp. 206–207

Chapter 3

Psychiatry

Isabel McMullen, Dinesh Bhugra,
and Gill McGauley

Mental health problems are estimated to affect one in four people each year in the UK, making mental illness one of the most common presentations to GP surgeries, outpatient clinics, and Emergency Departments. Yet many doctors and medical students feel uncertain about how to approach patients with a psychiatric disorder.

The key to becoming a good psychiatrist lies in the clinical interview. There are few physical signs or investigations that allow doctors to diagnose psychiatric illness, so a detailed history and mental state examination is important. As a psychiatrist, you are in the privileged position of having patients tell you their personal stories, and the skill is in listening attentively and asking relevant questions to help to clarify parts of the story. The best way to practise these techniques is to watch experienced clinicians at work, and to interview patients yourself.

Obviously diagnosis is important, so you need to be aware of the types of symptoms that fit with each type of disorder, as well as the medical conditions that may mimic psychiatric illness. Investigations may be necessary to rule out other diseases, and you need to be able to request these appropriately. Psychiatrists have access to a range of treatments—medical (e.g. antidepressants), psychological (e.g. cognitive behavioural therapy), and physical (e.g. electroconvulsive therapy)—and you need to know which ones to recommend. Most of these treatments are delivered in conjunction with the multidisciplinary team, so you should be clear about the roles of each team member.

Finally, there is overlap between psychiatry and the law, which can raise interesting ethical issues. It is sometimes necessary to treat a person against their will, for the safety of that person or others, so you need to know about mental health law. Psychiatrists are also often requested to provide a second opinion in difficult capacity assessments.

Isabel McMullen

QUESTIONS

Single Best Answers

1. A 53-year-old builder has injured his arm and is admitted to the ward. Late one night he becomes aggressive, shouting at the nurses and other patients, wanting to leave the ward, and saying that he can see ants running all over the walls. Which is the single most likely cause of these symptoms? ★

A Abnormal reaction to analgesic medication

B Alcohol withdrawal

C Dissocial personality disorder

D Head injury

E Past history of schizophrenia

2. A 20-year-old woman took 40 paracetamol tablets 9 hours ago. Which is the single most appropriate emergency treatment? ★

A Activated charcoal

B Diazepam

C Flumazenil

D *N*-Acetylcysteine

E Naloxone

3. A 34-year-old woman has severe abdominal pain and blood in her stool. Abdominal and pelvic examinations are normal, except for multiple surgical scars over the abdomen consistent with laparoscopies and an appendicectomy. She provides stool samples obtained at home that contain blood, but has not managed to produce one in hospital. Blood and urine investigations are normal, but she insists on further investigation and does not want to leave hospital. Which is the single most likely diagnosis? ★

A Delusional disorder

B Hypochondriacal disorder

C Malingering

D Mild–moderate depressive episode

E Munchausen syndrome

4. A 25-year-old man is disorientated and has slurred speech and respiratory depression. He also has miosis. Which is the single most likely cause? ★

A Alcohol abuse

B Carbon monoxide poisoning

C Opioid abuse

D Paracetamol overdose

E Salicylate overdose

5. A 36-year-old man goes to a plastic surgeon insisting on surgery, stating that his nose is too large and crooked. He says that people stare at him when he goes out, so he prefers not to leave the house. He attributes his recent job loss to his 'deformed nose.' He wears make-up to camouflage it, but would like surgery to correct what appears to be a normal nose. Which is the single most likely diagnosis? ★

A Body dysmorphic disorder

B Hypochondriasis

C Mild–moderate depressive episode

D Obsessive–compulsive disorder

E Social phobia

6. A 61-year-old man attends his GP at the request of his wife, who thinks he is drinking too much alcohol. Which single factor is a sign of alcohol dependence? ★

A A wide repertoire of alcoholic drinks

B Decreased alcohol tolerance

C Drinking 28 units of alcohol or more a week

D Drinking despite evidence of its harm to job and family

E Drinking until late in the evening

7. A 20-year-old man has a first episode of psychosis. Your consultant asks you to prescribe an atypical (or second-generation) antipsychotic. Which single drug should be prescribed? ★

A Chlorpromazine

B Haloperidol

C Lorazepam

D Mirtazapine

E Olanzapine

8. A 64-year-old man is recovering after a myocardial infarction (MI). His recovery is slowed by poor sleep, loss of appetite, lack of motivation, and feelings of hopelessness. Your consultant believes that he is depressed and asks you to commence antidepressant treatment. He has no other medical history. Which would be the single most appropriate class of drug to prescribe? ★

A Benzodiazepine

B Monoamine oxidase inhibitor (MAOI)

C Selective serotonin reuptake inhibitor (SSRI)

D Serotonin and noradrenaline (norepinephrine) reuptake inhibitor

E Tricyclic antidepressant

9. A 52-year-old woman has low mood, tiredness, and weight gain with decreased appetite. She is tearful and is overweight, with dry skin and thin hair. Which is the single most useful test to aid diagnosis? ★

A Chest X-ray

B ECG

C Full blood count

D Thyroid function tests

E Urea and electrolytes

10. A 35-year-old woman suddenly starts to feel dizzy and short of breath, with chest pains and a tingling sensation in her fingers. These symptoms worsen until she feels as if she is about to die. The episode lasts for about 10 minutes before resolving completely. Which is the single most likely diagnosis? ★

A Acute asthma

B Myocardial infarction

C Panic attack

D Temporal lobe epilepsy

E Transient ischaemic attack

11. A 36-year-old woman is 36 weeks pregnant with twins in England. She has obsessive–compulsive disorder. She is scheduled to have an elective Caesarean section for the delivery of her twins, due to complications in her last delivery and pre-eclampsia in this pregnancy. She has already consented to the operation. She has now become agitated and anxious and is refusing to cooperate, saying that she does not want to have the operation and wants to go home. Which is the single most appropriate course of action? ★

A Arrange emergency detention under the Mental Health Act 2007 (England and Wales), as her health depends on her being treated

B Assess her capacity to consent, and discuss the situation with a senior doctor

C Detain her for treatment, as she has a mental disorder as defined by the Mental Health Act 2007 (England and Wales)

D Prescribe sedative medication and advise the nurses to call when she is less agitated

E Tell the nurses to reassure her and carry on, as she has previously consented to the operation

12. A 44-year-old woman has taken an overdose of 20 paracetamol tablets. Which single factor indicates the highest risk of her going on to complete suicide? ★

A Having a psychotic illness

B Living with a partner

C Taking alcohol with the overdose

D Taking more than 50 tablets as an overdose

E Writing a suicide note before taking the overdose

13. A 58-year-old woman has gastritis. Her GP is concerned about her possible heavy use of alcohol, and arranges some screening questionnaires and blood tests. Which single result would indicate possible problem drinking or hazardous drinking? ★

A A decreased mean corpuscular volume (MCV)

B A low level of gamma-glutamyltranspeptidase (GGT)

C A score of 5 on the Alcohol Use Disorders Identification Test (AUDIT)

D One positive response on the CAGE questionnaire

E Raised urate levels

14. A 34-year-old man is brought to the Emergency Department by the police. He is agitated and elated. His blood pressure is 140/90 mmHg, his pulse rate is 120 bpm, and his pupils are dilated. Which single substance is he most likely to have been using? ★

A Cocaine

B Heroin

C Organic solvents

D Oxazepam

E Psilocybin

15. A 68-year-old man has a prominent impairment of recent memory with intact immediate recall. He has no evidence of generalized cognitive impairment and no impairment in his level of consciousness. Which is the single most likely diagnosis? ★

A Alzheimer's disease

B Delirium

C Korsakoff's syndrome

D Normal-pressure hydrocephalus

E Post-ictal state

16. A 74-year-old woman has bowel cancer being treated in England. The surgeons say that she requires surgery, which is potentially curative, and that without it she will die. The woman is refusing any surgical intervention. She had post-natal depression 42 years ago but is not currently suffering from any mental illness. Her present Mini-Mental State Examination (MMSE) score is 29/30. She knows about her diagnosis, believes that it applies to her, understands the risks and benefits of the proposed surgery, and is able to retain the information. Which is the single most appropriate course of action? ★

A Detain her under a section of the Mental Health Act 2007 (England and Wales) and perform the operation

B Discharge her from hospital

C Obtain a second opinion, and if that professional considers that the woman has capacity, comply with her wishes

D Restrain her under common law and perform the operation

E Use the Mental Capacity Act 2005 (England and Wales) to perform the operation

17. A 40-year-old woman is having intrusive and persistent thoughts that she is a 'dirty prostitute.' She recognizes that her thoughts are silly, but nevertheless feels ashamed of them. Although these thoughts get her down, she still enjoys life. Which is the single most likely diagnosis? ★

A Depressive disorder

B Generalized anxiety disorder

C Obsessive–compulsive disorder

D Psychotic episode

E Schizophrenia

18. A 28-year-old man is found in an alleyway in a semi-conscious state. He has a respiratory rate of 6 breaths/minute, a pulse rate of 50 bpm, and pinpoint pupils. Which is the single most appropriate drug to give? ★

A Clonidine

B Methadone

C Naloxone

D Naltrexone

E Thiamine

19. An 82-year-old man is forgetful, gets lost when he is out, and has difficulty finding his way home. On occasion he puts his keys in the microwave, and he does not appear to know how to use it to cook food. His memory problems seemed to get markedly worse around the time when he was admitted to hospital with a stroke 2 years ago, and again earlier this year when he could not speak for several minutes. His speech has since recovered. Which is the single most likely diagnosis? ★

A Alzheimer's disease

B Fronto-temporal dementia

C Lewy body dementia

D Normal ageing

E Vascular dementia

20. A 28-year-old woman has low mood and loss of appetite. She is still coping at work, but lacks energy and feels that her concentration is not as good as before. Her sleep is normal, and she enjoys spending time with her friends. She has never had any ideas of self-harm or suicide. Which is the single most appropriate course of action? ★

A Ask her to keep a mood diary and return to see you in 2 weeks' time

B Prescribe citalopram and see her again in 2 weeks' time

C Prescribe moclobemide and see her again in 4 weeks' time

D Refer her for cognitive behavioural therapy

E Tell her not to worry, and that it is normal to feel like this

21. A 29-year-old woman has recently been diagnosed as having generalized anxiety disorder. Which is the single best initial approach to management? ★

A Advise her to keep a diary of when she feels anxious

B Explain the condition to her, writing down the essential points

C Give her a standard information leaflet

D Provide her with information on the medication that can be used

E Recommend a self-help book

22. A 48-year-old man with alcohol dependence has been found wandering in the street. He has some clouding of consciousness, nystagmus, and ophthalmoplegia. Which is the single most appropriate medication to administer initially? ★

A Acamprosate

B Disulfiram

C Metoclopramide

D Naloxone

E Thiamine

23. A 30-year-old woman with panic disorder has been treated with cognitive behavioural therapy, which has only partially helped her symptoms. She requests further treatment and is prescribed citalopram. Which is the single most likely side-effect profile she should be warned about? ★

A Confusion and memory problems

B Drowsiness, palpitations, and postural hypotension

C Dry mouth, blurred vision, and constipation

D Nausea, gastrointestinal upset, restlessness, and insomnia

E Weight gain

24. A 28-year-old man who has recently been diagnosed with paranoid schizophrenia is started on risperidone. Which single common potential side-effect should he be advised about? ★

A Feeling more alert

B Gynaecomastia

C Hirsutism

D Improved sexual performance

E Weight loss

25. A 67-year-old man was diagnosed with dementia a year ago. He has previously been advised, both verbally and in writing, to inform the Driver and Vehicle Licensing Agency (DVLA) of his diagnosis. He says that he has not taken this advice, as he needs his car to get to the shops and to see his friends. The MMSE reveals that he is not disorientated but does show mild short-term memory loss. Which is the single most appropriate course of action? ★ ★

A Advise him again verbally that he needs to inform the DVLA

B Advise him verbally of your responsibility to disclose his diagnosis to the DVLA

C Advise him verbally that he should stop driving from now on

D Disclose his diagnosis to the DVLA

E Write to him again advising that he needs to inform the DVLA

26. A 20-year-old woman has panic attacks when she has to attend formal meetings at work. She also feels anxious when she meets her friends in the pub. Which is the single most likely diagnosis? ★ ★

A Adjustment disorder

B Generalized anxiety disorder

C Panic disorder

D Post-traumatic stress disorder

E Social phobia

27. A 60-year-old man asks for a repeat prescription for diazepam. He says that his GP started him on this treatment 3 months ago when he was anxious and depressed after losing his job. Which is the single most appropriate course of action? ★ ★

A Call his usual GP to arrange an appointment for him in 1 week's time

B Change his prescription to an antidepressant drug and explain that this would be a more appropriate treatment

C Explain that you cannot re-prescribe diazepam because of the risk of him becoming dependent

D Explain the risk of becoming dependent on diazepam and then re-prescribe diazepam at half the dose for 4 more weeks

E Explain the risk of becoming dependent on diazepam and then re-prescribe diazepam in a weekly decreasing dose

28. A 33-year-old woman with bipolar disorder is due to be started on a mood stabilizer. She has some questions about lithium. Which single symptom or sign is a common side-effect of lithium at therapeutic levels? ★ ★

A Coarse tremor

B Dysarthria

C Improvement of pre-existing skin conditions

D Thirst

E Weight loss

29. A 24-year-old man is found acting strangely in the park. He believes that MI5 are behind a plot to harm him, and are keeping him under surveillance. He hears himself being commented on by a voice 'reading the news', and thinks that his thoughts are being controlled by devices on buses. Which single symptom is one of Schneider's first-rank symptoms of schizophrenia? ★ ★

A Catatonia

B Ideas of reference

C Persecutory delusions

D Poverty of speech

E Third-person auditory hallucinations

30. A 26-year-old woman has emotional lability and a mildly depressed mood. She feels 'numb' and 'empty', and has recently often acted impulsively (e.g. by shoplifting). She uses recreational drugs regularly. She has no regular partner and is unemployed. She cuts herself in response to distressing feelings, but is not suicidal. Which is the single most likely diagnosis? ★ ★

A Antisocial personality disorder

B Avoidant personality disorder

C Emotionally unstable personality disorder

D Histrionic personality disorder

E Mild depressive episode

31. A 79-year-old man has personality change and worsening orientation. He has a tremor, extensor plantar reflexes, and bilateral small pupils that do not constrict in response to light but do constrict on accommodation. Which is the single most useful diagnostic investigation? ★

A Chest X-ray

B CT scan of the brain

C EEG

D MRI of the brain

E Venereal Disease Research Laboratory (VDRL) test

32. The police bring a 23-year-old man to the Emergency Department, who they have detained because he was standing in the middle of the road shouting at the traffic and threatening to stab drivers. The doctor is asked to take a history and examine the patient. Which is the single most appropriate initial action for the doctor to take? ★

A Arrange for the interview to take place in a quiet, private room

B Ask the police to be present during the interview

C Remove from the room any sharp items that could be used as weapons

D Talk to the police about the patient's presentation and behaviour

E Tell another member of staff to note down where the interview will take place

33. The wife of a patient is in a distressed state. She tells her GP that her husband is wandering around the house at night and that she is afraid to sleep in case he accidentally harms himself. She says that he has already drawn up a Personal Welfare Lasting Power of Attorney (LPA), which is registered at the Office of the Public Guardian, and that he has appointed her as his 'attorney' to make decisions on his behalf. The GP knows that the patient has a diagnosis of dementia, although it is 6 months since he last saw him. The patient's wife asks the GP to prescribe some sedative medication, adding that her husband is quite happy to take a tablet at night. Which is the single most appropriate response for the GP to make? ★ ★ ★

A Advise the patient's wife that he would need to talk to other members of the family as well before he prescribed any medication

B Explain to the patient's wife that an LPA does not cover decisions about medical treatment

C Explain to the patient's wife that he would need to see her husband to assess whether he lacks the capacity to decide whether or not to take sedative medication

D Explain to the patient's wife that she cannot give consent on behalf of her husband for him to prescribe medication

E Prescribe a small dose of sedative medication for the patient and see him in 1 week

34. A 23-year-old woman has had psychological and somatic symptoms of anxiety for 3 weeks, which mostly occur when she has to drive her car in the city. This is the first time she has suffered from these symptoms. Which is the single most appropriate treatment? ★ ★ ★ ★

A Anxiety management training

B Behavioural therapy

C Brief psychodynamic psychotherapy

D A selective serotonin reuptake inhibitor (SSRI)

E A tricyclic antidepressant

35. A 3-year-old boy has been referred to the paediatrician and child psychiatrist for assessment. He was late in starting to talk, and is falling behind his peers at nursery. He is thought to have mild learning disability. His parents have some questions. Which single statement about mild learning disability is appropriate when counselling the parents? ★ ★ ★ ★

A A specific cause cannot be identified in 50% of cases

B Epilepsy occurs in 70% of people with mild learning disability

C Fragile X syndrome is an X-linked recessive condition that can cause mild learning disability

D Only a very small number of people with mild learning disability are capable of working in adulthood

E The expected IQ range is between 20 and 35

36. A 6-year-old boy does not talk and will not play with other children. He is only interested in toy cars, and lines them up in a particular order. His teacher says that he cannot read or write like the other children, and that he has temper tantrums for no obvious reason. Which is the single most likely diagnosis? ★ ★ ★ ★

A Asperger's syndrome

B Autism

C Normal child

D Obsessive–compulsive disorder

E Rett's syndrome

37. A 30-year-old man with paranoid schizophrenia has not responded to two consecutive 8-week trials of olanzapine and risperidone at therapeutic doses. Which is the single most appropriate course of action? ★ ★ ★ ★

A Combine olanzapine and risperidone

B Commence clozapine

C Commence haloperidol

D Commence risperidone long-acting injection

E Continue olanzapine at a higher dose

38. A 35-year-old man was prescribed an antidepressant 8 months ago for a moderately severe depressive episode. This was his first depressive episode. He now feels that he has almost recovered, and wants to know when he can stop taking the antidepressant. Which is the single most appropriate piece of advice? ★ ★ ★ ★

A He must take the tablets for the rest of his life

B He should continue the medication for 1 to 2 months after he has recovered

C He should continue the medication for 4 to 6 months after he has recovered

D He should continue the medication for 1 year after he has recovered

E He should stop the antidepressants immediately if he feels that he is back to normal

39. A 30-year-old man with paranoid schizophrenia on the ward becomes very agitated one night. He is pacing around, talking to himself, and appears to be responding to hallucinations. He is verbally aggressive and hostile to staff and other patients. He has a history of violence when unwell. Simple de-escalation techniques have failed to calm the situation, but he is willing to take medication. Which is the single most appropriate management? ★ ★ ★ ★

A Give clozapine 50 mg orally and review in 1 hour

B Give haloperidol 10 mg IM and review in 1 hour

C Give lorazepam 2 mg orally and review in 1 hour

D Give olanzapine 20 mg IM and review in 1 hour

E Request police presence on the ward

40. A 31-year-old single mother discloses that she regularly cuts herself in front of her 6-year-old son, and that he often becomes distressed if he thinks she is feeling sad. She is not taking him to school every day. Which is the single most appropriate course of action? ★ ★ ★ ★

A Contact the school to find out whether her son's teacher has any concerns about him, and document the discussion

B Find out whether she has any extra support, such as a family member, who could come and help her to look after her son

C Inform the police and social services immediately

D Speak to a senior colleague and the designated child protection lead at the trust

E Tell her that if she does not stop self-harming in front of him, you will have to take action

41. A 22-year-old woman has recurrent depressive episodes. Her main symptoms are low mood, anhedonia, insomnia, and weight loss secondary to poor appetite. She has had adverse reactions to selective serotonin reuptake inhibitors (SSRIs) in the past. Which would be the single most appropriate medication to prescribe? ★ ★ ★ ★

A Citalopram

B Fluoxetine

C Mirtazapine

D Paroxetine

E Sertraline

42. A 47-year-old man with paranoid schizophrenia has been known by his mental health team for 15 years. He has needed eight admissions during that time. He has recently deteriorated due to non-compliance with medication, and is threatening his neighbours with violence. He is now in a very similar state to that with which he has presented in the past when unwell. He is refusing to agree to admission to hospital for treatment. Which is the single most appropriate section of the Mental Health Act 2007 (England and Wales) to use? ★ ★ ★ ★

A Section 2

B Section 3

C Section 5

D Section 17

E Section 136

43. A 48-year-old woman is admitted to hospital for routine surgery. She takes once-daily lithium for treatment of bipolar disorder. Which is the single correct time to take her blood to check plasma levels of lithium? ★ ★ ★ ★

A Immediately before her dose

B 2 hours after her dose

C 8 hours after her dose

D 12 hours after her dose

E 20 hours after her dose

44. A 35-year-old man who is opiate dependent is considering tackling his addiction. In discussing treatment options, which is the single most appropriate piece of advice to include? ★ ★ ★ ★

A Methadone has a shorter half-life than heroin

B Naltrexone is an opiate agonist, and is an alternative to methadone

C Opiate withdrawal results in death if untreated

D Opiate withdrawal causes restlessness, abdominal pain, and anxiety

E The withdrawal syndrome will begin 2 to 3 days after heroin was last taken

45. A previously healthy 78-year-old man has a severe depressive illness. He has not responded to various treatments so far, and his consultant wants to prescribe a tricyclic antidepressant. Which is the single most important investigation before commencing treatment? ★ ★ ★ ★

A CT scan of the brain

B ECG

C Full blood count

D Urea and electrolytes

E Urinalysis

Extended Matching Questions

Causes of confusional states

For each patient, choose the *single* most likely diagnosis from the list of options below. Each option may be used once, more than once, or not at all. ★

A Alcoholic hallucinosis

B Alzheimer's disease

C Delirium

D Delirium tremens

E Depressive disorder

F Depressive pseudodementia

G Dissociative fugue

H Schizophrenia

I Subdural haematoma

J Vascular (multi-infarct) dementia

K Wernicke's encephalopathy

1. A 45-year-old man has become confused and disorientated. He was seen in the Emergency Department 3 days ago and was treated for a head injury that he sustained in a fight after a night of heavy drinking.

2. A 78-year-old woman has become confused, scared, and agitated on the ward. Urinalysis shows the presence of protein and blood.

3. A 55-year-old man with chronic alcohol abuse is agitated and disorientated. He spent yesterday in the pub but has not been able to buy a drink since. He is sweating profusely and appears frightened.

4. A 65-year-old man with diabetes, ischaemic heart disease, and hypertension has had memory impairment for 6 months. His wife says that he occasionally gets confused at night.

5. A 60-year-old homeless woman is brought to the Emergency Department. She smells of alcohol, is confused, and has nystagmus and a broad-based, staggering gait.

Alcohol and drug misuse

For each clinical situation, choose the *single* most likely treatment approach from the list of options below. Each option may be used once, more than once, or not at all. ★

A Acamprosate

B Buprenorphine

C Chlordiazepoxide

D Diazepam

E Disulfiram

F Fluoxetine

G Haloperidol

H Parenteral thiamine

I Olanzapine

J Oral methadone

6. A 60-year-old man who is dependent on alcohol experienced a seizure when he was previously detoxified. He wants to undergo a further detoxification.

7. A 25-year-old man has been smoking cannabis for 6 months. He has started to become suspicious of colleagues, believing that they are spying on him, and that they can overhear his thoughts.

8. A 50-year-old man has successfully completed an alcohol detoxification programme and starts to develop cravings for alcohol. He does not want to engage in 'talking therapies.'

9. A 45-year-old man is currently dependent on alcohol and wants to undergo outpatient detoxification.

10. A 55-year-old man with alcohol dependence is acutely confused and has ophthalmoplegia.

Causes of memory loss

For each patient, choose the *single* most likely diagnosis from the list of options below. Each option may be used once, more than once, or not at all. ★

A Alzheimer's disease

B Creutzfeldt–Jakob disease

C Depressive pseudodementia

D Huntington's disease (chorea)

E Korsakoff's syndrome

F Lewy body dementia

G Mild cognitive impairment

H Parkinson's disease

I Pick's disease

J Vascular (multi-infarct) dementia

11. An 85-year-old man has an isolated memory impairment. He scores 26/30 on the MMSE, and his activities of daily living are unimpaired.

12. A 62-year-old man is forgetful. He cannot remember how he got to the surgery, but is able to recall an address on testing of his memory. He has gynaecomastia and palmar erythema.

13. A 70-year-old woman is convinced that her neighbours are stealing her food. She has become increasingly forgetful over the last year, but blames others when she cannot find things. She wanders at night, thinking it is daytime, and finds it difficult to button up her clothes.

14. A 73-year-old woman has had memory loss for 3 months, which is worse in the morning. She is distressed by her symptoms, but responds to most questions by saying 'I don't know.'

15. A 57-year-old woman has had failing memory and a tremor of her right hand for 3 years. She is finding it harder to keep up with her husband when out walking, and has difficulty getting out of chairs and up the stairs of the bus.

Causes of severe behavioural disturbance

For each patient with disturbed behaviour, choose the *single* most likely diagnosis from the list of options below. Each option may be used once, more than once, or not at all. ★

A Acute psychotic episode

B Delusional disorder

C Emotionally unstable personality disorder

D Mania with psychotic features

E Normal grief

F Psychotic depression

G Schizoaffective disorder

H Schizophrenia

I Schizotypal personality disorder

16. A 21-year-old man has been hearing voices for 2 days, which he believes belong to the FBI agents who are following him. He is scared because he thinks the FBI wants him dead, so is unable to sleep. He has no psychiatric or medical history. He uses cannabis most days, and 3 days ago he took what his friends think was cocaine at a party.

17. A 43-year-old woman believes that her husband is about to leave her because she is a useless wife and mother. She is convinced that he is having an affair and that his family are 'against her.' She now feels that her GP is part of the plot to help him to divorce her. She says that she has failed and deserves to be punished. Over the past few months she has become increasingly withdrawn and neglectful of her personal hygiene. She sleeps poorly and has lost weight. She suffered with post-natal depression after the birth of her son 5 years ago.

18. A 50-year-old man has had ideas about the police wanting to harm him for 20 years. He has a vast collection of evidence that this is the case, including his post being delivered late on significant days, silent phone calls, his water supply being 'poisoned', and a sign going up that is an anagram of his name. He has never experienced any auditory or visual hallucinations.

19. A 23-year-old woman is troubled by voices. These are a combination of derogatory comments about her and remarks about the abuse that she suffered as a child. The voices do not sound real, but often feel like her own thoughts being echoed aloud. She finds them distressing and copes by drinking alcohol or cutting herself.

20. A 29-year-old man has been hearing voices for the last 5 years that provide a running commentary on his actions and tell him how to live his life. He has recently started to communicate with his grandmother, who died 2 years ago, and believes that he is carrying out her wishes. He believes that doctors are able to hear his thoughts, and he therefore dislikes them. He does not trust people who wear red, as he thinks they are part of the 'Devil's Army.'

Causes of anxiety

For each patient, choose the *single* most likely diagnosis from the list of options below. Each option may be used once, more than once, or not at all. ★ ★

A Acute stress disorder

B Agoraphobia

C Dysthymia

D Generalized anxiety disorder

E Panic attack

F Panic disorder

G Paranoid personality disorder

H Post-traumatic stress disorder

I Simple phobia

J Social phobia

21. A 22-year-old woman has recurrent 20-minute episodes during which she fears that she is going to die because her heart races, she has chest pain and difficulty breathing, and she feels dizzy, nauseous, and shaky. The episodes occur in a variety of situations, and she spends much of her life fearing the next episode.

22. A 35-year-old woman has overwhelming worries about every-day matters, and is unable to relax. She feels on edge all the time, although she has periods when the anxiety becomes worse and she feels dizzy and has palpitations, shortness of breath, and hot flushes.

23. A 32-year-old woman becomes very anxious in a variety of situations—for example, at the supermarket or on public trans-port. She has shortness of breath, feels sweaty, and is fearful that she may collapse in public. As a result, she rarely leaves the house alone.

24. A 42-year-old soldier is unable to relax and has been irritable since returning from conflict 5 months ago. His concentration is poor and he has problems falling asleep. He has vivid memories of a car bomb attack in which some of his regiment died, and he now avoids driving a car if at all possible.

25. A 27-year-old man has few friends and tries to avoid contact with people because he is worried that this will end in humilia-tion. He does not believe that he has anything to add to social gatherings, and he thinks that people laugh at him behind his back. When he finds himself in such situations, he becomes sweaty, blushes, and suffers from a dry mouth and trembling.

Causes of learning disability

For each patient with learning difficulties, choose the *single* most likely diagnosis from the list of options below. Each option may be used once, more than once, or not at all. ★ ★

A Angelman's syndrome

B Down's syndrome

C Fetal alcohol syndrome

D Fragile X syndrome

E Klinefelter's syndrome

F Lesch–Nyhan syndrome

G Prader–Willi syndrome

H Rett's syndrome

I Tuberous sclerosis

J Turner's syndrome

26. A 5-year-old girl showed normal development until the age of 2 years, but now has epilepsy and episodes of limb spasticity. She has involuntary hand flapping and hand wringing. Her personality has changed and she is irritable and anxious at times. Her intellectual abilities have also deteriorated, and she now has a severe learning disability.

27. A 3-year-old girl with fair hair and a prominent jaw has epilepsy and severe learning disability. She is unable to walk properly due to jerky limb movements. She has episodes of uncontrollable laughter and hand flapping.

28. A 39-year-old man with lifelong short stature and moderate learning disability starts to experience difficulty in daily tasks, such as cooking, that he would previously have been able to perform easily. His language skills are deteriorating, and he has become more withdrawn and irritable.

29. A 3-year-old girl has short stature and low weight with micro-cephaly, a short palpebral fissure, and a smooth philtrum. She was late to walk and talk, and is falling behind her peers at playgroup.

30. A 16-year-old man has moderate learning disability and epilepsy. He has a long face with large ears, and has hyperextensible joints in his fingers. He is anxious in company, and has few friends and a rigid style of communicating.

Multidisciplinary teams

For each patient, choose the *single* most useful member of the multidisciplinary team from the list of options below. Each option may be used once, more than once, or not at all. ★ ★ ★

A Benefits adviser

B Community psychiatric nurse

C Consultant psychiatrist

D Occupational therapist

E Physiotherapist

F Psychologist

G Social worker

H Specialty registrar psychiatrist

I Staff nurse

J Support worker

31. A 26-year-old woman has recently been diagnosed with paranoid schizophrenia after several admissions to hospital. She has been discharged, but there is concern that she does not fully understand or accept the implications of her diagnosis and may stop taking her medication. She needs regular support and education about her illness and relapse prevention.

32. A 37-year-old man with paranoid schizophrenia has been admitted to a rehabilitation ward. His positive symptoms are well controlled by the medication that he is taking, but he has problems with motivation and activities of daily living. He has particular difficulties with regard to shopping and cooking for himself, and in attending to his personal hygiene. He would like some help to learn how to do these things.

33. A 45-year-old father of two children has severe recurrent depressive episodes that have required hospitalization. He is unable to work for long periods of time, but is hopeful that he may return to part-time employment in the future. However, he is starting to experience financial difficulties because he does not receive any financial support, and he finds the filling in of application forms complicated.

34. A 35-year-old woman with bipolar affective disorder is singing loudly late into the night, and has been seen in the street wearing very few clothes and conspicuous make-up. She is throwing out large items of furniture and is trying to give her neighbours' children her money and jewellery, saying that she wants to 'spread her wealth.' She requires a review of her mental state with a view to possible admission.

35. A 42-year-old man with obsessive–compulsive disorder is worried because his symptoms have worsened recently. He says that he is compliant with his medication, but he has recently lost his job. His wife is concerned that he does not seem 'his usual self', and she is worried that there might be 'something else going on.' He needs a review.

ANSWERS

Single Best Answers

1. B ★ OHCS 9th edn → pp. 350–351

Alcohol withdrawal can cause delirium tremens, which is characterized by florid visual or tactile hallucinations, typically of small creatures. This is relatively common in drinkers who are suddenly admitted to hospital, and a detailed alcohol history should always be taken to try to prevent withdrawal using appropriate medication.

→ http://guidance.nice.org.uk/CG115

2. D ★ OHCS 9th edn → p. 192

All patients who have a delayed presentation (more than 8 hours) after paracetamol overdose should have N-acetylcysteine started immediately.

3. E ★

In Munchausen syndrome, or factitious illness, affected individuals fake illness in order to gain medical attention. Often, reasonably serious symptoms, such as blood in the stools or urine, can be falsified. These cannot be reproduced when the person is being directly observed. Malingering is the term used for people who feign illness for another gain (e.g. financial benefit or avoidance of work). Hypochondriasis refers to an excessive worry about illness, and these patients may often have vague medical symptoms such as palpitations or abdominal pain.

4. C ★ OHCS 9th edn → p. 362

These are the classic signs of acute opioid intoxication.

5. A ★

The key here is that the person is excessively concerned with an imagined abnormality in his physical appearance, which is affecting his life. It is not an obsession and is not affecting mood. The social withdrawal is occurring because of the concern about the feature, rather than because of anxiety. Hypochondriasis is a fear of serious illness, rather than concern about physical features.

6. D ★ OHCS 9th edn → p. 363

It is not the amount drunk, or the quality of what a person drinks, but the effect that it has on their life that characterizes dependence.

7. E ★   OHCS 9th edn → p. 360

Olanzapine is a commonly used atypical antipsychotic drug. These have different side-effects from typical antipsychotic drugs, such as haloperidol and chlorpromazine. Lorazepam is a benzodiazepine. Mirtazapine is an antidepressant.

8. C ★   OHCS 9th edn → p. 340

Depression following MI is associated with a poor prognosis, although the evidence that treatment of depression improves this is equivocal. Tricyclic antidepressants increase the risk of MI, so they should not be used in patients with ischaemic heart disease. SSRIs may have a protective effect. Benzodiazepines do not treat depression. MAOIs are used only rarely for depression nowadays, due to their potentially lethal interactions.

Anon. (2008). Depression, antidepressants and heart disease. *Drug Ther Bull* **46**: 29–32.

9. D ★   OHCS 9th edn → p. 336

Hypothyroidism is a recognized cause of depression, and it also causes physical symptoms, including lethargy, weight gain, constipation, dry skin and hair, and oedema. Recognition of these symptoms should point towards investigation of thyroid function to guide appropriate treatment.

10. C ★   OHCS 9th edn → p. 344

Although some of these symptoms may occur in any of the options given, the young age, combination of symptoms, and complete resolution within a short time make a panic attack the most likely diagnosis.

11. B ★   OHCS 9th edn → pp. 402–403

Although this woman has signed a consent form, a patient can withdraw consent at any time. Although she has a history of obsessive–compulsive disorder, which would satisfy the definition of a mental disorder under the Mental Health Act 2007 (England and Wales) or the Mental Health (Care and Treatment) (Scotland) Act 2003, she cannot be detained under the Act to allow medical or surgical treatment to continue. The fact that she has pre-eclampsia does not constitute a danger to herself or others (i.e. her babies) under the Act, as this risk is not arising from her mental disorder.

12. A ★   OHCS 9th edn → p. 338

→ www.medicine.manchester.ac.uk/mentalhealth/research/suicide/prevention/nci/

(Key findings (suicide) from the National Confidential Inquiry into Suicide and Homicide by People with a Mental Illness)

13. C ★   OHCS 9th edn → p. 363

A raised MCV and GGT are indicative of problem drinking. Two or more positive responses are needed on the CAGE questionnaire. Urate levels are raised in about 50% of all people with drinking problems, but they are only useful as screening tests for men, as they are poor discriminators in women. AUDIT is a simple 10-question test developed by the World Health Organization (WHO) to determine whether a person's alcohol consumption may be harmful. The test was designed to be used internationally, and was validated in a study using patients from six countries. Questions 1 to 3 deal with alcohol consumption, Questions 4 to 6 relate to alcohol dependence, and Questions 7 to 10 consider alcohol-related problems.

→ http://whqlibdoc.who.int/hq/2001/WHO_MSD_MSB_01.6a.pdf

14. A ★

Cocaine abuse has sympathomimetic effects, and causes tachycardia, hypertension, and pupillary dilatation. Heroin has the opposite effect. Solvent abuse causes signs similar to those of alcohol intoxication, but may also include hallucinations. Psilocybin, which is found in 'magic mushrooms', also causes hallucinations. Oxazepam is a benzodiazepine.

15. C ★

In delirium and in a post-ictal state, there would be alteration in the level of consciousness. In Alzheimer's disease, the person would have generalized cognitive impairment that is progressive. Normal-pressure hydrocephalus usually presents with a triad of ataxia, dementia, and urinary incontinence.

16. C ★   OHCS 9th edn → p. 403

The Mental Capacity Act 2005 (England and Wales) provides a statutory framework to empower and protect vulnerable people who are not able to make their own decisions. It is underpinned by five key principles:

1. Every adult is presumed to have capacity unless it is proven otherwise.
2. Individuals must be supported to make their own decisions.
3. Individuals retain the right to make what might be viewed as unwise or eccentric decisions.
4. Any action taken on behalf of individuals who lack capacity must be done in their best interests.
5. Any action taken on behalf of people who lack capacity must be the least restrictive option.

In this case, the patient has capacity and is not suffering from any mental impairment (e.g. psychotic depression or dementia). Therefore, although it seems an unwise decision, she has the right to refuse surgery. However, in complicated and life-threatening cases such as this, it is always wise to seek a second opinion, and if necessary to involve your trust's legal department. Note that Scotland has a separate legal framework, the Adults with Incapacity (Scotland) Act 2000.

→ www.direct.gov.uk/en/DisabledPeople/HealthAndSupport/
YourRightsInHealth/DG_10016888

→ www.scotland.gov.uk/Publications/2003/03/16933/21228

17. C ★   OHCS 9th edn → p. 346

An obsession is a stereotyped, purposeless word, idea, or phrase that comes into the mind and that originates from the person, rather than from outside. The patient realizes that it is not true.

18. C ★

Bradypnoea, bradycardia, and pinpoint pupils strongly suggest opioid overdose. The treatment for this is intramuscular and intravenous naloxone.

19. E ★   OHCS 9th edn → pp. 350–351, 648, 650

The history of strokes, together with the progressive dementia, points to vascular dementia caused by multiple infarcts. Alzheimer's disease is a possibility, but the vascular history suggests otherwise. Lewy body dementia is characterized by hallucinations, visuo-perceptual defects, and a fluctuating course. Frontotemporal dementia, or Picks's disease, is characterized by frontal lobe signs such as disinhibition.

20. A ★   OHCS 9th edn → p. 336

In mild depression, watchful waiting and review is the first-line strategy. Although this woman has low mood and lack of energy, she is functioning at work and socially, and has no physical symptoms and no suicidal ideation.

→ http://guidance.nice.org.uk/CG90

21. B ★   OHCS 9th edn → p. 344

All of these approaches could be used, but as anxiety disorders are maintained by fears about the nature and consequences of symptoms, an explanation of the condition is the first step in treatment. Anxious patients do not concentrate well, especially when given new information. Therefore writing down the key points so that the patient can read them at home is the optimum approach.

22. E ★

Chronic alcohol consumption can result in thiamine deficiency due to inadequate nutritional intake, impaired uptake in the bowel, and impaired metabolism. Thiamine deficiency can lead to alcohol-induced brain damage, so thiamine should be replaced intravenously if patients with alcohol abuse show signs of possible brain damage. The other medications have roles in treating various addictions, but are not appropriate in this case.

23. D ★   OHCS 9th edn → p. 340

All of the other side-effect profiles are prominent in patients who are prescribed tricyclic antidepressants. Confusion is more likely to occur in elderly patients who are prescribed tricyclic antidepressants, and this together with signs such as dry mouth is due to the anticholinergic effects of these drugs. Their adrenergic antagonism may cause cardiovascular effects. Citalopram is a selective serotonin reuptake inhibitor (SSRI).

24. B ★   OHCS 9th edn → pp. 360–361

Risperidone is an atypical antipsychotic and is associated with hyperprolactinaemia. This may result in gynaecomastia and galactorrhoea in men, and disturbance of the menstrual cycle in women. The side-effects of risperidone sometimes include sexual dysfunction and weight gain.

25. E ★ ★

The General Medical Council (GMC) has clearly stated that, for several conditions (including dementia), doctors should not only advise patients of the possibility of having to stop driving, but should also take steps to ensure that the relevant statutory authorities are informed of breaches of regulation if there is reasonable concern about public safety. Initially this should be done by informing the patient of the need to let the DVLA know about their condition. The fact that this patient is not disorientated, his short-term memory loss is mild, and he was only diagnosed a year ago would suggest that you do not have to make an immediate clinical decision that he is unfit to continue driving until the DVLA has assessed him.

Breen DA, Breen DP, Moore JW, Breen PA and O'Neill D (2007). Driving and dementia. *BMJ* **334**: 1365–1369.

Harris M (2000). Psychiatric conditions with relevance to fitness to drive. *Adv Psychiatr Treat* **6**: 261–269.

→ http://apt.rcpsych.org/content/6/4/261.full

General Medical Council (2004). *Confidentiality: protecting and providing information.*

→ www.gmc-uk.org/guidance/current/library/confidentiality.asp

Driver and Vehicle Licensing Agency. *At a Glance Guide to the Current Medical Standards of Fitness to Drive.*

→ www.dvla.gov.uk/medical/ataglance.aspx/

26. E ★ ★   OHCS 9th edn → p. 344

There are many different types of anxiety disorder. The fact that all of the patient's symptoms occur in social situations makes social phobia the most likely diagnosis.

27. E ★ ★   OHCS 9th edn → p. 368

Long-term use of benzodiazepines runs the risk of creating dependency. However, suddenly stopping them may cause a withdrawal syndrome. If this man has run out of diazepam, there is a risk that he will develop withdrawal syndrome if he has to wait a week to see his usual GP. Antidepressants will not help the withdrawal. A reducing regime can be used to wean him off the diazepam, but this should be supervised.

28. D ★ ★   OHCS 9th edn → p. 354

Lithium has a narrow therapeutic index, which means that the difference between effective and toxic doses is small. Thirst is a common side-effect. Fine tremor is also common, and weight gain and skin rash can occur. At toxic levels, dysarthria can occur.

29. E ★ ★   OHCS 9th edn → p. 358

Schneider's first-rank symptoms of schizophrenia are symptoms that, if present, are strongly suggestive of schizophrenia. They include the following:

- auditory hallucinations: hearing thoughts spoken aloud, hearing voices referring to oneself in the third person, auditory hallucinations in the form of a commentary
- thought withdrawal, insertion, and interruption
- thought broadcasting
- somatic hallucinations
- delusional perception
- feelings or actions experienced as being generated or influenced by external agents.

30. C ★ ★   OHCS 9th edn → p. 366

There are a number of personality disorders, each of which has its own unique features. They all start in childhood or late adolescence, and are patterns of inner experience and behaviour that remain stable throughout life and are different from that which would normally be expected in the society in which the person lives. There are two types of emotionally unstable personality disorder—borderline and impulsive. In the borderline type, the person tends to form intense relationships and to have rapid fluctuations in mood, with impulsivity, disturbed self-image, recurrent self-harm, and chronic feelings of emptiness.

31. E ★

Neurosyphilis is an uncommon cause of psychiatric illness, but is suggested by the Argyll Robertson pupils as described in the question. These are a highly specific sign of neurosyphilis.

32. D ★

Careful consideration has to be given to team safety when assessing potentially dangerous patients. The police may know the patient and be able to provide valuable information, such as a history of mental health problems or drug use. In addition, the information that the doctor is given by the police may well influence how and where the patient is seen. For example, it may become clear that the doctor needs to be accompanied by another healthcare professional. The police may well have to leave, and their information should be sought early. Although a quiet, private room may help to calm the patient, it may put the doctor in a dangerous situation. Any room that is used should have all potentially dangerous objects removed from it, and the doctor should always place him- or herself between the door and the patient. Although having the police present for the interview may seem a sensible option, it will compromise confidentiality, and if the patient has paranoid thoughts or beliefs, a police presence may well exacerbate these. It is better to ask a member of the healthcare staff whether there is a need for the doctor to be accompanied.

33. C ★★★

Under the Mental Capacity Act 2005 (England and Wales), a Personal Welfare LPA does not come into effect until the patient has lost capacity to consent, even though it may be registered with the Office of the Public Guardian. As the GP has not seen the patient for 6 months, he does not know whether he has capacity to decide for himself whether to take medication. Although he has a diagnosis of dementia, which may have affected his capacity under the Act, every adult has the right to make their own decisions and must be assumed to have capacity to make them unless it is proved otherwise. Until the GP has assessed the patient, he cannot assume that he does not have capacity. If the GP has assessed the patient and has judged that he does lack capacity to decide whether to take this medication, and that prescribing such medication is in his best interests, then the Personal Welfare LPA would allow his wife to give or refuse consent to the administration of treatment by a person providing healthcare. Note that a separate act, the Adults with Incapacity (Scotland) Act 2000, is in place in Scotland.

→ www.direct.gov.uk/en/Governmentcitizensandrights/
Mentalcapacityandthelaw/index.htm

→ www.scotland.gov.uk/Topics/Justice/law/awi

34. A ★ ★ ★ ★   OHCS 9th edn → p. 344

Anxiety management training is a form of cognitive behavioural therapy that has the best record for the treatment of anxiety. Behavioural therapy with graded exposure to anxiety-provoking stimuli may be useful in some specific cases. Paroxetine (an SSRI) can help to treat social anxiety, but non-pharmacological measures should be tried first.

35. A ★ ★ ★ ★   OHCS 9th edn → p. 364

More often than not a cause cannot be identified, although genetic causes should be considered, as they may have implications for genetic counsel-ling. Fragile X syndrome is not X-linked recessive, but is caused by an expansion of triplet repeats on the X chromosome through successive generations. Epilepsy can occur in learning disability, but only in about 30% of individuals. There is a spectrum of learning disability, and many adults will be able to be supported in finding suitable employment. In mild learning disability, the expected IQ is approximately 50–70, in moderate learning disability it is 35–50, and in severe learning disability it is 20–35. However, IQ provides no information about individual strengths and weaknesses, so it is not the best way of classifying learning disability.

36. B ★ ★ ★ ★   OHCS 9th edn → p. 394

These are all features that suggest a diagnosis on the autistic spectrum. Autism is a pervasive developmental disorder with features that include the following:

- impaired communication: in the most severe cases there is no lan-guage at all, no imaginative play, and echolalia (repeating other people's words)
- impaired social interaction (e.g. not responding to other people's emotions)
- restricted, repetitive, and stereotyped patterns of movement, behav-iours, and interests (e.g. liking rigid routines and becoming upset when these do not occur, enjoying activities such as lining toys up or spinning wheels repeatedly)
- onset before the age of 3 years.

Asperger's syndrome is classified by some as being at one end of the spectrum. However, language is retained in Asperger's syndrome, although it is qualitatively different. Rett's syndrome occurs in girls.

37. B ★ ★ ★ ★   OHCS 9th edn → p. 360

In England and Wales there are published guidelines on the use of cloza-pine in the treatment of resistant schizophrenia:

→ http://guidance.nice.org.uk/CG82

38. C ★★★★

If antidepressants are stopped too soon, about 50% of patients will relapse. Antidepressants should be withdrawn over a period of several weeks.

→ http://guidance.nice.org.uk/CG90

39. C ★★★★   OHCS 9th edn → p. 359

You should familiarize yourself with your local trust's rapid tranquilliza-tion policy for cases such as this. In general, start with simple de-escalation techniques (talking calmly, using non-hostile body language, etc.), and if necessary offer oral medication first, only moving on to intramuscular administration if the patient refuses oral treatment. A benzodiazepine such as lorazepam is a good starting point, and you should review the situation regularly. If this is not effective, an antipsychotic should be pre-scribed. First-generation antipsychotics such as haloperidol are no longer the first-line approach, because of the risk of dystonic side-effects. Olanzapine would be an appropriate choice, but note that it cannot be given within 1 hour of lorazepam.

40. D ★★★★

In the interest of safeguarding children, concerns like this should not be ignored. According to recommendations from *Good Medical Practice*, all doctors have a duty to consider the interests of children who may be in the care of adult patients. There are local systems in place to discuss non-urgent concerns, and all trusts will have a designated lead for child protection.

→ www.gmc-uk.org/Child_protection_consultation__2_.pdf_42123624. pdf

41. C ★★★★   OHCS 9th edn → p. 340

Fluoxetine, paroxetine, sertraline, and citalopram are all SSRIs. For patients who cannot tolerate SSRIs, the next choice would be mirtaza-pine, which is a reuptake inhibitor and receptor blocker that affects the levels of noradrenaline (norepinephrine) and serotonin in the synapses.

→ http://guidance.nice.org.uk/CG90

42. B ★★★★   OHCS 9th edn → p. 400

The Mental Health Act 2007 applies to England and Wales. Scotland has a separate Act—the Mental Health (Care and Treatment) (Scotland) Act 2003.

- Section 2 is a (maximum) 28-day section for assessment of a patient with a mental disorder. It is used if the diagnosis is not clear.
- Section 3 is a (maximum) 6-month section for treatment. It is only used if the patient is well known to the healthcare professionals and the symptoms are consistent with the type that they suffer from when unwell.

- Section 5 is an emergency holding power, used by nurses (Section 5(4)) or doctors (Section 5(2)) to detain an informal patient who is already an inpatient.
- Section 17 is the part of the Mental Health Act that allows the Responsible Clinician to grant a detained inpatient leave from the hospital.
- Section 136 is an emergency section used by the police to bring a person in a public place whom they suspect is suffering from a mental disorder to a place of safety in order that they may be assessed.

→ www.legislation.gov.uk/ukpga/2007/12/contents

→ www.scotland.gov.uk/Publications/2008/09/24090333/1

43. D ★★★★ OHCS 9th edn → p. 354

→ www.bnf.org (Registration required)

44. D ★★★★ OHCS 9th edn → p. 362

Opiate withdrawal is an unpleasant experience, but does not result in death in healthy individuals. Symptoms include restlessness, anxiety, insomnia, abdominal pain, nausea, diarrhoea, yawning, and piloerection. Methadone is a long-acting opiate, with a long half-life, which is taken orally once a day and so reduces the 'rush' that is caused by injecting heroin. Naltrexone is an opiate antagonist that can be used after completing detoxification, to reduce the risk of relapse.

45. B ★★★★ OHCS 9th edn → p. 340

Tricyclic antidepressants can slow cardiac conduction and may cause arrhythmias and heart block. This is particularly dangerous in the elderly, in whom the side-effect of postural hypotension may also be a problem.

Extended Matching Questions

1. I ★

Subdural haematomas commonly occur after head injuries. In alcoholics, the injury need only be quite minor. A subacute subdural haematoma typically presents 3 to 7 days after the injury, and causes a variety of symptoms, including headache, confusion, nausea, and weakness.

2. C ★

Delirium is acute confusion, with onset over a period of hours or days. It is common in the elderly when they are in hospital for a number of reasons. Urinary tract infection, as indicated by the abnormal urinalysis, is a common cause. Delirium tremens refers specifically to delirium caused by withdrawal from alcohol.

3. D ★

Delirium tremens is common and should not be forgotten. See Single Best Answer 1.

4. J ★

There are many causes of dementia. In patients with risk factors for vascular disease, multi-infarct dementia should be considered. It is caused by multiple infarcts in the brain. These may have been silent strokes, without overt clinical signs.

5. K ★

General feedback on 1–5: OHCS 9th edn → pp. 350–351

6. D ★

Benzodiazepines are commonly used to help to relieve symptoms of alcohol detoxification and to prevent life-threatening complications such as seizures. Chlordiazepoxide has a slower onset of action, and most seizures occur within 48 hours of stopping alcohol, so diazepam is used in cases where complications are expected. Diazepam should be given under close supervision.

7. I ★

This man has features of a psychosis, probably secondary to the drug misuse. Olanzapine is an atypical antipsychotic, so it causes fewer side-effects than typical antipsychotics such as haloperidol.

8. A ★

This drug is thought to reduce the cravings for alcohol by stabilizing the imbalance of neurotransmitters in the brain. Disulfiram can also be used in alcoholics, but this works by causing an acute sensitivity to alcohol when the person drinks, and will not alter their cravings.

9. C ★

Chlordiazepoxide is the first-line treatment in uncomplicated detoxification programmes used at home.

10. H ★

This man has signs of Wernicke's encephalopathy, caused by acute, severe thiamine deficiency in alcoholics.

General feedback on 6–10: OHCS 9th edn → pp. 363, 513

11. **G** ★

Although the MMSE alone should not be used to make diagnoses in iso-lation, it is the most commonly used screening tool for cognitive func-tion. Scores of 25–30 are essentially normal. Coupled with the isolated memory problem and unimpaired activities of daily living, this indicates only a mild impairment.

12. **E** ★

Korsakoff's syndrome is part of a spectrum of brain damage caused by lack of thiamine in the brain in alcoholics. It causes memory loss, vision changes, incoordination, and hallucinations, to varying degrees. The clues here that distinguish this from other forms of memory impairment are the other signs of alcoholic liver disease. Alcohol abuse should always be considered in patients with memory impairment.

13. **A** ★

This is an enduring, progressive deficit of memory and cognition. In the early stages there is amnesia and spatial disorientation, while in the later stages the personality deteriorates. There are no neurological abnor-malities here and no evidence of other disease, which makes the other options less likely.

14. **C** ★

In the elderly, depression is a common cause of memory and functional impairment and should always be screened for. This woman's low mood and poor responses and the short time period involved make depression likely.

15. **H** ★

Parkinson's disease affects the substantia nigra and reduces the amount of dopamine neurotransmitter, which in turn affects signals to the mus-cles. The main symptoms are slowness of movement (bradykinesia), stiff-ness of muscles (rigidity), and tremor.

General feedback on 11–15: OHCS 9th edn → pp. 350–353

16. **A** ★

Drug abuse is a common cause of acute psychotic episodes, especially in young people.

17. **F** ★

Depression can also have psychotic symptoms. It is important to screen for and recognize depression, as this will alter management.

18. B ★

Delusions are fixed, false beliefs. They can occur as part of schizophrenia, but other symptoms would also need to be present. This man has an isolated delusion.

19. C ★

This is characterized by impulsive behaviour and lack of self-control, together with disturbances of self-image, unstable relationships, feelings of emptiness, and recurrent self-harm. This woman is not hearing voices outside herself, which means that these are not auditory hallucinations as seen in psychosis.

20. H ★

This man has hallucinations, delusions, and thought broadcasting that have been evident for more than 6 months.

General feedback on 15–20: OHCS 9th edn → pp. 356–358

21. F ★★

Panic disorder has both physical and psychological symptoms. These are typical of the physical symptoms and are affecting the patient psychologically. Panic disorder is characterized by recurrent, severe panic attacks and behavioural change associated with these. Thinking about the attacks may bring one on.

22. D ★★

Generalized anxiety disorder is characterized by excessive, uncontrollable, and often irrational worry about everyday things in a disproportionate way. It interferes with the activities of daily living.

23. B ★★

This is a specific anxiety disorder characterized by fear of having a panic attack in a public place. Because of this fear, individuals with this disorder do not leave the house alone. The trigger may be unfamiliar environments, open spaces, or crowds.

24. H ★★

The clear history of a traumatic event is the clue here. In post-traumatic stress disorder there is an ongoing reaction to the psychological trauma, and symptoms such as flashbacks, nightmares, and hyperarousal occur.

25. J ★★

These anxiety symptoms are specific to social situations.

General feedback on 20–25: OHCS 9th edn → pp. 344–346

26. H ★★

Rett's syndrome has an X-linked dominant pattern of inheritance, so it only affects girls. There is typically a history of developmental regression (i.e. loss of skills). One of the characteristic features seen in Rett's syndrome is repetitive hand movements. This syndrome is the second most common cause of severe learning disability in girls. Genetic testing can be undertaken.

27. A ★★

This is caused by a deletion in the maternally inherited chromosome 15 (a deletion in the paternally inherited chromosome 15 causes Prader–Willi syndrome). Children with Angelman's syndrome have characteristic jerky movements and hand flapping, which led to the old-fashioned term 'happy puppet syndrome'. They also have severe epilepsy that can be difficult to control. Genetic testing can be undertaken.

28. B ★★

Down's syndrome is now usually diagnosed at birth or at least within the first year of life. However, some older patients may not have been diagnosed, and are recognized by the characteristic dysmorphic features such as short stature and facial and hand features. There are varying degrees of learning disability in Down's syndrome, and many patients can live semi-independently. As people with Down's syndrome get older they are at increasing risk of developing Alzheimer's disease, which usually starts in their thirties.

29. C ★★

The severity of this syndrome depends on the level of alcohol consumption in pregnancy. There may not be a clear history of alcohol consumption. Babies are usually small for dates and have microcephaly, as alcohol affects brain development. They have characteristic facial features, which may be subtle, including a hypoplastic upper lip with an absent philtrum (groove), and small eyes with a short palpebral fissure. They have global developmental delay and learning disabilities.

30. D ★★

Fragile X syndrome describes a pattern of inheritance on the X chromosome with triplet repeats that lengthen as they are transmitted from one generation to the next. At a critical size, the repeats become unstable and cause problems. Both girls and boys can be affected, but boys are more severely affected because of the lack of a second X chromosome. Often there is a history of mild learning difficulty in the mother and learning difficulty in other male relatives. Boys with fragile X syndrome have characteristic features, including large ears and facial asymmetry, and may be on the autistic spectrum. Fragile X syndrome is the commonest inherited form of learning disability.

General feedback on 26–30: OHCS 9th edn → pp. 138, 352, 648

31. **B** ★ ★ ★

Many patients need ongoing support after discharge, and it is vital to consider this and to make sure that adequate team support is in place. The role of the community psychiatric nurse is to be a point of contact in the community, to support patients through difficult times, to support the family, to help with medication, and to check that patients remain well.

32. **D** ★ ★ ★

Occupational therapists are skilled in assessing the impact of illness on daily life, and they help to ensure that patients can undertake all of the activities of daily living.

33. **A** ★ ★ ★

Mental illness can have a serious impact on financial well-being for the patient and the whole family, and patients are often unaware of the financial support to which they may be entitled. A benefits adviser can provide help with accessing benefits and filling in forms.

34. **C** ★ ★ ★

The consultant psychiatrist is best placed to facilitate admission and liaise with all of the necessary team members. This woman may need to be admitted under the Mental Health Act, so an approved psychiatrist is needed to facilitate this.

35. **H** ★ ★ ★

The trainee is also a vital member of the team and can see patients on the wards and in clinics.

General feedback on 30–35: → www.rcpsych.ac.uk/mentalhealthinfo/treatments/communityteams.aspx

Ophthalmology

Venki Sundaram

Ophthalmology principally aims to prevent visual loss, restore visual function, and relieve ocular discomfort. The majority of the pathology can be directly visualized, and thus requires proficient ocular examination techniques and visual recognition skills.

Another distinguishing aspect of ophthalmology is the overlap between medical and surgical conditions. Common systemic diseases such as diabetes and hypertension have ocular features, and diseases involving every organ of the body can have ocular manifestations. A thorough medical knowledge is paramount, as is the ability to collaborate with other medical teams. Intraocular surgery for conditions such as cataract is technically challenging, as ocular tissues are so delicate. It therefore requires high levels of fine hand–eye coordination.

As an ophthalmologist you will be faced both with acute eye conditions, some of which are sight-threatening and require prompt diagnosis and management, and with chronic conditions, which require monitoring and treatment for many years. You will be exposed to patients of all ages, from premature babies to the elderly, so good communication with a wide range of patient groups and their families is essential. Patients often say that what they fear most is losing their sight. Therefore empathy and support for patients with debilitating visual impairment are imperative.

The questions in this chapter will test your knowledge of acute emergency ophthalmic presentations and the understanding and interpretation of ophthalmic examination, as well as ocular conditions that have systemic associations. In addition, questions relating to ophthalmic risk factors, communication, and probity are included. Eye problems can be daunting to many medical students and doctors. Through practice in examining patients and recognizing key conditions, confidence can be gained in how best to manage these patients and, importantly, when to refer them to other specialties.

QUESTIONS

Single Best Answers

1. A 72-year-old man has painless, sudden of loss of vision in his right eye. Twenty-four hours later, visual acuity in his right eye is limited to counting fingers, and there is a carotid bruit on the right side. His BP is 155/100 mmHg. His fundus appearance is shown in Plate 4.1 (see Colour Plate section). Which is the single most likely diagnosis? ★

A Central retinal artery occlusion

B Central retinal vein occlusion

C Papilloedema

D Rhegmatogenous retinal detachment

E Transient ischaemic attack

2. A 69-year-old woman with hypermetropia has had increasing left ocular pain, redness, and blurring of vision for 6 hours. She is seeing haloes around bright lights, and she feels nauseous. Her left eye is shown in Plate 4.2 (see Colour Plate section). Which is the single most likely diagnosis? ★

A Acute angle closure

B Anterior scleritis

C Bacterial conjunctivitis

D Iritis

E Subconjunctival haemorrhage

3. A 72-year-old woman has sudden loss of vision in her right eye. She has been experiencing temporal headache, jaw ache, and shoulder pain for the last 2 weeks. Her visual acuity in the right eye is limited to seeing hand movements. The appearance of her fundus is shown in Plate 4.3 (see Colour Plate section). Which single investigation would be most likely to support the diagnosis? ★

A Blood cultures

B CT scan of the head

C Erythrocyte sedimentation rate (ESR)

D Full blood

E Fluorescein angiography

4. A 54-year-old woman has had increasing severe right ocular pain for 3 days, which is now affecting her sleep. Her vision is unaffected but she has considerable ocular tenderness. Her right eye is shown in Plate 4.4 (see Colour Plate section). Which single systemic condition is most commonly associated with her ocular condition? ★

A Acute lymphocytic leukaemia

B Bacterial endocarditis

C Multiple sclerosis

D Malignant carcinoma of the colon

E Rheumatoid arthritis

5. A 6-year-old boy has had increasing fever, malaise, and right lid swelling over the last 48 hours. His eyelid is shown in Plate 4.5 (see Colour Plate section). When the eyelid is opened with difficulty, he has conjunctival chemosis and mild proptosis, with limitation of upgaze. His temperature is 38.6°C. Which is the single most appropriate treatment? ★

A Intravenous broad-spectrum antibiotics

B Oral antihistamines

C Oral broad-spectrum antibiotics

D Systemic steroids

E Topical antibiotics

6. A 22-year-old man is hit in his right eye with a glass bottle. His vision is 6/24 unaided, and his eye is shown in Plate 4.6 (see Colour Plate section). Which is the single most serious complication of this injury? ★

A Cataract

B Endophthalmitis

C Hyphaema

D Iridodialysis

E Lens subluxation

7. A 27-year-old woman has accidentally splashed an alkaline detergent in both eyes. She is in considerable discomfort and has marked diffuse bilateral conjunctival injection and hazy corneas. Which is the single most appropriate immediate management? ★

A Application of eye pads

B Irrigation with normal saline

C Limbal stem-cell transplant

D Topical antibiotic

E Topical vitamin C

8. A 33-year-old man has had increasing diplopia, drooping of the left upper lid, and headache over the last 2 days. There is a complete left ptosis and the left pupil is dilated. The left eye is depressed and abducted, and eye movements are limited in all directions except downgaze and abduction. Which single condition must be investigated for immediately? ★

A Aponeurotic ptosis

B Myasthenia gravis

C Orbital myositis

D Posterior communicating artery aneurysm

E Thyroid eye disease

9. A 77-year-old woman had uneventful right cataract surgery 3 days ago. She now has increasing pain, redness, and reduced vision in this eye. Her vision is 6/60, and there is marked conjunctival injection and anterior chamber inflammation with a 1-mm hypopyon. The fundal view is hazy. Which is the single most likely diagnosis? ★

A Acute angle-closure glaucoma

B Bacterial conjunctivitis

C Bacterial endophthalmitis

D Iritis

E Scleritis

10. A 45-year-old woman complains of irritable eyes and double vision when she looks to her side. She is concerned that her facial appearance has changed in recent months, and that she has had some weight loss despite an increased appetite. There is moderate conjunctival vessel injection, and the sclera is visible between her upper lids and cornea. There is proptosis of both eyes. On extreme lateral gaze there is limitation of eye movement and diplopia. Which is the single most likely cause of her eye problems? ★

A Carotid-cavernous fistula

B Optic nerve glioma

C Orbital haemangioma

D Orbital myositis

E Thyroid eye disease

11. A 66-year-old man who smokes 15 cigarettes a day has unequal pupil size. His visual acuity is unaffected and his right pupil is smaller, becoming more apparent in darker conditions. His pupils react normally to light and there is mild right upper lid ptosis. Which is the single most appropriate test to confirm the diagnosis of his pupil abnormality? ★ ★

A Chest X-ray

B ESR

C MRI scan of the head

D Topical cocaine eye drops

E Topical phenylephrine eye drops

12. A 47-year-old man is referred after being found on annual check-up by his optician to have raised intraocular pressures. He has type 2 diabetes and his uncle is on treatment for glaucoma. His visual acuity is 6/6 in both eyes with glasses for myopia, and his intraocular pressures are 34 mmHg in the right eye and 36 mmHg in the left eye. Which single risk factor is most important for the development of glaucoma? ★ ★

A Age

B Diabetes

C Family history of glaucoma

D Myopia

E Raised intraocular pressure level

13. A 41-year-old woman has had gradual visual loss in her left eye over the last few years. Her optician initially commented that she had an early cataract that was too 'immature' for surgery to be considered, but this has now progressed. Her visual acuity is 6/60 in the left eye and 6/6 in the right eye. There is a mild left cortical cataract, and fundal examination reveals a total rhegmatogenous retinal detachment. Which is the single most appropriate course of action? ★ ★

A Explain in detail the pathological processes involved in developing a retinal detachment

B Explain that she has developed a retinal detachment, and discuss the surgical options for reattaching the retina, and the likely visual prognosis

C Explore why she did not suspect that something more serious was causing her visual loss

D Recommend that she pursues legal action against her optician for delay in diagnosis of a retinal detachment

E Tell her that she has a retinal detachment and is likely to go blind in the left eye, but that she still has the sight in her other eye

14. A 68-year-old woman with hypertension has had gradually decreasing vision in her left eye. Her visual acuity is 6/36, improving to 6/9 with pinhole testing, in this eye. Which is the single most likely diagnosis? ★ ★ ★

A Cataract

B Central retinal artery occlusion

C Central retinal vein occlusion

D Dry age-related degeneration

E Glaucoma

15. A 58-year-old man with hypertension who has previously undergone a renal transplant complains of floaters and blurring of vision in his right eye. He is highly myopic, and his visual acuity is 6/18. Fundoscopy shows peripheral areas of yellow-white retina, surrounded by haemorrhage. Which is the single most likely diagnosis? ★ ★ ★

A Central retinal vein occlusion

B Choroidal melanoma

C Cytomegalovirus retinitis

D Hypertensive retinopathy

E Retinal detachment

16. A 65-year-old woman with multiple sclerosis has reduced right visual acuity. She has type 2 diabetes, and underwent squint surgery to her right eye as a child. Her right visual acuity is 6/36 with glasses, and there is no pinhole improvement. A swinging flashlight test shows a right relative afferent pupillary defect. Which is the single most likely diagnosis? ★ ★ ★ ★

A Amblyopia

B Background diabetic retinopathy

C Cataract

D Diabetic macular oedema

E Optic neuritis

17. A 73-year-old man had routine right cataract surgery 2 weeks ago. At his post-operative visit it was found that his vision is not as clear as he was expecting. Refraction and review of the operation notes reveal a significant (4 dioptre) refractive error due to an intraocular lens of the wrong power being inserted during surgery. Which is the single most appropriate course of action? ★ ★ ★ ★

A Advise the patient that things will settle and that it can take time for the brain to adjust to the new vision

B Apologize and explain that an error has occurred, and involve a senior colleague who can discuss the various management options

C Apologize and explain that the wrong lens was inserted during the operation because the surgeon was handed a lens of the wrong power

D Apologize and explain that some natural lens fragments have unfortunately been retained in the eye and that a further operation is needed to remove these and replace the lens

E Do not mention that an error has occurred, and advise the patient to visit his optician, who can 'fine-tune' his vision

Extended Matching Questions

Causes of visual loss

For each patient with visual loss, choose the *single* most likely diagnosis from the list of options below. Each option may be used once, more than once, or not at all. ★

A Anterior ischaemic optic neuropathy

B Branch retinal vein occlusion

C Cataract

D Central retinal artery occlusion

E Central serous retinopathy

F Choroidal neovascular membrane

G Demyelinating optic neuritis

H Diabetic macular oedema

I Diabetic vitreous haemorrhage

J Dry age-related macular degeneration

K Primary open-angle glaucoma

L Retinal detachment

1. A 31-year-old woman has had increasing visual loss in her right eye over the last 3 days, and ocular discomfort on eye movement. She has had several episodes of leg weakness in the last 6 months.

2. A 56-year-old man with type 2 diabetes has a sudden reduction of vision in his left eye. The fundal view is poor with ophthalmoscopy, and B-scan ultrasonography shows no retinal detachment.

3. A 72-year-old woman has had increasing difficulty reading over the last 2 years. She has had previous bilateral cataract surgery, and fundal examination shows bilateral macular drusen, atrophy, and pigmentary changes, with no retinal fluid.

4. A 45-year-old man with type 2 diabetes and myopia has loss of vision in the inferior half of his right visual field. There are retinal flame-shaped haemorrhages with vessel tortuosity along the superior vascular arcade.

5. A 67-year-old man has had worsening of central vision in his right eye over the last week. There is a submacular greyish lesion on the fundus with subretinal oedema and haemorrhage.

ANSWERS

Single Best Answers

1. **A**
OHCS 9th edn → p. 435

A pale fundus with a 'cherry-red' spot at the macula is classically found in central retinal artery occlusions. Hypertension and sources of potential emboli (e.g. carotid artery disease) are risk factors for developing this condition.

2. **A** ★
OHCS 9th edn → p. 430

Ocular pain and nausea are due to the acute rise in intraocular pressure. This also causes corneal oedema with reduced vision and glare symptoms. Examination findings are typically ciliary vessel injection, mid-dilated pupil, shallow anterior chamber depth, and high intraocular pressure (> 40 mmHg). Increasing age and hypermetropia are risk factors for developing acute angle closure.

3. **C** ★
OHCS 9th edn → p. 434

This woman has a left anterior ischaemic optic neuropathy, secondary to giant-cell arteritis (temporal arteritis). A very raised ESR is typically found, and patients can experience temporal headache, jaw pain, and myalgia. The posterior ciliary arteries may be affected by the arteritis, resulting in an anterior ischaemic optic neuropathy causing dramatic visual loss and a swollen disc with flame-shaped haemorrhages.

4. **E** ★
OHCS 9th edn → p. 448

This woman has a right diffuse anterior scleritis. This is associated with an underlying autoimmune condition in nearly 50% of cases, of which rheumatoid arthritis is the most common.

5. **A** ★
OHCS 9th edn → p. 420

This boy has a right-sided orbital cellulitis, which usually arises from bacterial spread from adjacent sinuses. This differs from preseptal cellulitis, as congestion from orbital spread results in chemosis, proptosis, and restriction of eye movement, in addition to eyelid involvement. This is an emergency, requiring urgent IV antibiotics and possible drainage of any sinus abscess. A delay in treatment can result in complications such as optic nerve compression and meningeal spread.

6. B ★   OHCS 9th edn → p. 452

This man has a penetrating eye injury. This requires urgent closure of the corneoscleral laceration, with appropriate antibiotic cover. A delay in management can increase the risk of developing endophthalmitis, and can result in severe, permanent visual loss.

7. B ★   OHCS 9th edn → p. 452

Alkali-induced eye injuries are potentially sight-threatening, as they can cause liquefactive necrosis of ocular tissue. Immediate copious irrigation with normal saline until a neutral pH is reached can prevent further alkali penetration and destruction.

8. D ★

This man has a left-sided third-nerve palsy. Pupil involvement implies a compressive cause, and the rapid, painful onset suggests an expanding lesion such as a posterior communicating artery aneurysm. This needs to be investigated immediately in order to prevent a potentially fatal sub-arachnoid haemorrhage.

9. C ★   OHCS 9th edn → p. 442

Post-operative bacterial endophthalmitis is a rare but serious complica-tion of cataract surgery. Patients typically present with poor vision, pain, and significant intraocular inflammation within 2 weeks of surgery. The fundal view can be obscured by significant vitritis. Prompt recognition and management can help to prevent irreversible visual loss.

10. E ★

This woman has thyroid eye disease, which can cause ocular irritation, conjunctival vessel injection, and lid retraction. Proptosis and restriction of eye movements are secondary to enlargement of the extraocular mus-cles. The other conditions typically result in unilateral proptosis and are not associated with systemic symptoms.

11. D ★★   OHCS 9th edn → p. 424

This man has right-sided Horner's syndrome. This occurs because of interrupted sympathetic innervation to the eye. Topical 4% cocaine drops instilled into both eyes will only cause dilatation of the normal pupil. This is because cocaine blocks the reuptake of noradrenaline (norepine-phrine) at nerve endings, causing pupil dilatation. In Horner's syndrome, no noradrenaline is secreted, so cocaine has no effect. Horner's syn-drome has many causes, including Pancoast tumours of the lung.

12. E ★★   OHCS 9th edn → p. 440

Raised intraocular pressure is the strongest risk factor for the development and progression of glaucoma. Lowering of intraocular pressure is currently the only method of preventing visual field loss.

National Institute for Health and Clinical Excellence (2009). *Glaucoma: diagnosis and management of chronic open angle glaucoma and ocular hypertension:*

→ www.nice.org.uk/CG85

13. B ★★★

The news that this woman's visual loss is the result of retinal detachment rather than cataract is likely to come as a shock and be anxiety-provoking. Therefore this information needs to be conveyed in a sensitive manner without placing the blame on either the patient or other professionals. Attention can then be focused on the management options available, including what possible surgery would involve and the likely visual outcome.

14. A ★★★   OHCS 9th edn → p. 442

Pinhole use focuses light entering the eye, so can compensate for refractive errors (up to several dioptres) or conditions that cause glare, such as cataract. Visual acuity improvement with pinhole testing therefore implies a refractive problem rather than an organic problem.

15. C ★★★

Cytomegalovirus (CMV) retinitis usually only affects immunocompromised individuals. It results in areas of yellow-white retinal necrosis and haemorrhage ('pizza-pie' appearance), which can spread if not recognized and promptly treated. A raised brown fundal mass is usually evident with choroidal melanoma. Although central retinal vein occlusion can also cause retinal haemorrhage, retinal necrosis is not a feature. Significant retinal haemorrhage and retinal necrosis do not occur with retinal detachment or hypertensive retinopathy.

16. E ★★★★   OHCS 9th edn → p. 434

A relative afferent pupillary defect occurs when light shone into the affected eye causes initial dilatation of both pupils. The pupils initially dilate because the stimulus from light being shone into the affected eye is less than the stimulus of withdrawing light from the unaffected eye. This most commonly occurs in optic nerve lesions, but can also be due to other gross pathology of the anterior visual pathway (e.g. total retinal detachment, optic tract lesions).

17. B ★ ★ ★ ★

For a variety of reasons, insertion of an intraocular lens of the wrong power during cataract surgery can unfortunately occur. Patients have a right to know about this, and need to be appropriately informed of such errors and the various management options, so that they can make an informed decision on how best to rectify any visual difficulties.

The surgeon who performs the operation is ultimately responsible for the power of the intraocular lens that is inserted, even if they are handed the wrong one by a scrub nurse or assistant.

Careful pre-operative selection, double-checking of the correct lens power, and the surgeon him- or herself obtaining the correct lens from the lens storage area can help to ensure that the correct lens is inserted.

Extended Matching Questions

1. G ★

Multiple sclerosis is a demyelinating disease that can affect the optic nerve and cause optic neuritis. The distinct episodes of weakness are caused by demyelination of peripheral nerves.

2. I ★

A sudden reduction of vision with a poor fundal view in diabetic patients implies a vitreous haemorrhage due to proliferative diabetic retinopathy. B-scan ultrasonography can be useful for excluding large retinal tears or detachment as the cause of the vitreous haemorrhage.

3. J ★

Gradual visual loss (especially difficulty with reading) is typical of dry age-related macular degeneration. Both eyes are usually affected, with macular drusen, atrophy, and retinal pigment epithelial changes being seen.

4. B ★

This produces haemorrhage and vessel tortuosity in the region of the affected vessel. This can cause corresponding visual field loss (i.e. inferior field loss in superior occlusions) as retinal images are inverted.

5. F ★

Choroidal neovascular membranes can appear as greyish lesions beneath the macula. Leakage of blood or fluid from the membrane usually results in a fairly acute onset of central visual loss due to photoreceptor damage.

General feedback on 1–5: OHCS 9th edn → pp. 434–439

Chapter 5

Primary care

Philippa Edwards, Will Coppola,
and Kamila Hawthorne

GPs are the gatekeepers of the National Health Service in the UK, and virtually all referrals to secondary care are made through them. The breadth and depth of the discipline can at times seem overwhelming, although the old adage 'common things occur commonly' still holds. GPs need to be confident in the diagnosis and management of conditions from birth to the grave, and to know their boundaries of competence and when to refer to secondary care. The complexity of the GP consultation includes the following two points:

1. Many conditions present in a relatively undifferentiated form to the GP, whose job it is to try to identify whether the condition is normal or abnormal, and whether it is serious or minor.

2. GPs develop a close professional relationship with many of their patients, and may also be the point of contact for other members of the family, neighbours, and friends of the patient. This knowledge is an important aspect of their holistic approach to medicine, and is much valued by their patients. As the nineteenth-century physician, Sir William Osler (1849–1919), said, '*The good physician treats the disease; the great physician treats the patient who has the disease.*'

The commonest presentations to GPs in the UK are for respiratory problems, chronic disease management, musculoskeletal disorders, and psychological problems. Health promotion, in particular smoking cessation and the management of obesity, is also important in preventing chronic illness. Although many presentations are minor and self-limiting, serious illnesses also occur, and GPs need to be able to recognize them, sometimes in the early stages.

The questions in this chapter will assess your knowledge in the common areas that present, testing diagnostic skills and reasoning. They also test negotiating skills to ensure patient compliance, teamworking within the primary care setting, and risk management.

Kamila Hawthorne

QUESTIONS

Single Best Answers

1. A 26-year-old woman has registered as a new patient, and her New Patient Health Check reveals a body mass index (BMI) of 32 kg/m^2. Which is the single best explanation to the patient of what BMI means? ★

A It is a measure of cardiovascular risk

B It is a measure of how much weight a person needs to lose

C It is a representation of weight for height

D It is a way of calculating how fat the body is

E It is the ratio of hip circumference to waist circumference

2. A 44-year-old builder has acute low back pain following heavy lifting at work the previous day. He is finding it difficult to walk. Which single feature of his presentation would warrant urgent referral to hospital? ★

A Difficulty in passing urine

B Inability to perform a straight leg raise beyond 20°

C Pain down the back of both legs

D Reduced ankle jerks

E Use of inhaled steroids for his asthma

3. The mother of a 16-year-old girl is worried that her daughter is becoming depressed, and she knows that the girl came to see you last week. The daughter's behaviour at home has been deteriorating, and there have been a lot of arguments. The mother wants to know what the recent consultation was about and to seek your opinion about what to do. Which is the single most appropriate course of action? ★

A Advise her that she can apply to the primary care trust for access to her daughter's medical record

B Do not discuss her concerns about her daughter at all, as the daughter is over 16 years of age

C Listen to her concerns but do not reveal information about the daughter, as the daughter has not given you consent

D Tell her a little about the recent consultation and ask her to come back later with her daughter

E Tell her what transpired in the recent consultation, as she has a right to know as a parent

4. A 65-year-old man has had a previous small myocardial infarction. He wants advice on modifying his risk factors to prevent further health problems. Which is the single most important modifiable risk factor for stroke in this patient? ★

A Alcohol intake of 40 units per week

B Atrial fibrillation

C Body mass index of 35 kg/m²

D Previous myocardial infarction

E Raised blood pressure of 165/105 mmHg

5. A 44-year-old businessman has recently been diagnosed with high blood pressure. He does not want to take any medication. Which is the single best approach to take in the consultation to try and come to a resolution? ★

A Allow him to do what he wants to do, but tell him that he will have to see another doctor in the future

B Be friendly towards him, so that he is more likely to come back if he changes his mind

C Identify and consider his viewpoint, bringing this into the decision-making process

D Tell him all about the different medications and their side-effects so that he has all of the information

E Tell him that he needs to take the medication which has been chosen for him or he may be at risk of harm

6. A 35-year-old woman is unable to sleep, is tired during the day, and is having problems at work as a result. Which single aspect of her history is the most likely to have a significant bearing on her presenting complaint? ★

A She drinks about 20 units of alcohol per week

B She has a 9-year-old daughter

C She has a stressful job as a teacher

D She is tearful and cannot concentrate

E She smokes 10 cigarettes a day

7. A 17-year-old girl is going away to college next year. She is seek-
ing information about the human papilloma virus (HPV) vaccine, as
she missed the programme at school and is now considering having the
vaccination. Which is the single most appropriate piece of information to
give her about the vaccine? ★

A If she has already had sexual intercourse, she has probably already
been exposed to HPV and it is not worth having the vaccination

B If she has the vaccination, it will protect her against HPV and she will
not need cervical smear testing later in life

C If she suffers from eczema or asthma, she will not be able to have the
vaccination because of the risk of severe allergic reactions

D The vaccination is only available as part of a primary immunization
course for infants, and she is too old to be included in the 'catch-up'
cohort

E The vaccination is 99% effective in preventing cervical abnormalities
caused by HPV types that can lead to cervical cancer, and she is
eligible to have it

8. A 52-year-old woman wants advice about mammography breast
screening before her appointment. She has read a newspaper art-
icle which suggests that it may not be valuable and could even be potentially harmful. You are not aware of this evidence and have not seen any
recent literature on the subject. Which is the single most appropriate
response to give in this situation? ★

A Advise her that there is a financial penalty for practices if patients do
not attend screening appointments, so she should make every effort
to keep her appointment

B Agree with her that there are reasonable concerns about the benefits
of mammography, and advise her not to take any further part in the
screening programme

C Explain that you are not aware of the evidence that she has raised
with you, so you are going to refer her to a specialist breast surgeon
for up-to-date advice

D Explain that you are not aware of the evidence that she has raised
with you, but that you could help her to interpret it once you have
looked at it yourself

E Explain that you are not aware of the evidence that she has raised
with you, so it is unlikely to be true and she should attend for
screening

9. A 48-year-old woman has recently moved into the practice area. At her induction health check, the practice nurse notes that her weight is 85 kg and her height is 160 cm. Which single health factor would you consider in advising her about her weight? ★

A She is at increased risk of stomach cancer and needs to lose weight to a BMI of 25 kg/m^2 to bring her risk down to acceptable levels

B She is at increased risk of stomach cancer and needs to lose 20 kg to bring her risk down to acceptable levels

C She is at increased risk of hypertension and should lose 5 kg to bring her risk down to acceptable levels

D She is at increased risk of kidney stones and needs to lose 10 kg to bring her risk down to acceptable levels

E She is at increased risk of type 2 diabetes and should lose 20 kg to bring her risk down to acceptable levels

10. A 22-year-old student has muscle aches, malaise, headache, and anorexia that started 2 days ago. Today he has a temperature of 39.4°C. Which is the single most important direct question to ask him as part of history taking in order to confirm the likely diagnosis? ★

A Has he been bitten by an animal recently?

B Has he had close contact with anyone else with similar symptoms?

C Has he recently eaten any food that he thinks might have 'gone off'?

D Has he travelled overseas recently?

E Is he taking any medication at present?

11. A 55-year-old diabetic man asks for the vaccines he had last year against flu and pneumonia. His records show that he had the influenza and pneumococcal vaccines last year. Which is the single most appropriate piece of advice to give him? ★

A The influenza vaccine that he had last year will protect him against influenza for another 5 years

B He does not need another influenza vaccine this year but should have it next year

C He does not need another pneumococcal vaccine this year but should have it next year

D He is in a high-risk category for influenza and should have this vaccine every year

E He is in a high-risk category for pneumonia and influenza and should have both vaccines every year

12. A 50-year-old man with convictions for violence comes to the surgery reception smelling of alcohol and demanding dihydrocodeine. Which is the single best way of managing this situation? ★

A Ask him to take a seat in the waiting room to be seen in order with the other patients

B Immediately show him to the next available doctor

C Phone the police and ask them to remove him

D Physically eject him from the premises and lock the surgery door

E Place him in a vacant room and ask a doctor to see him when they are available

13. An 84-year-old woman is in hospital recovering from a total hip replacement following a fall in her flat. She was previously independent, despite living on the first floor, and drove her own car to the nearby shops. Who is the single best professional to ensure that she is safe to return to her flat? ★

A Age Concern worker

B GP

C Health visitor

D Occupational therapist

E Physiotherapist

14. An 18-year-old man has a sore throat, fever, and malaise. A monospot test is sent and comes back positive. Which is the single most important element to avoid at this stage? ★

A Alcohol

B Contact sports

C Fatty foods

D Kissing

E Paracetamol

15. A 21-year-old student comes for a repeat prescription of her combined oral contraceptive pill (the Pill). She has been having bad one-sided headaches with flashing lights lasting a few minutes prior to the headache since starting the Pill. She has a past history of migraine when stressed, and has some exams coming up. Her blood pressure is 100/70 mmHg and her clinical examination is normal. Which is the single most appropriate management? ★

A Advise her that the headaches are most probably caused by exam stress

B Advise her to stop taking the Pill if the flashing lights last longer than 60 minutes

C Stop the Pill she is taking and try a different combined oral contraceptive pill

D Stop the Pill she is taking and consider a progestogen-only pill instead

E Stop the Pill she is taking and refer her urgently to a neurologist

16. A 65-year-old woman, who lives alone, has chronic knee pain and is prescribed a course of non-steroidal anti-inflammatory drugs (NSAIDs) for the first time. After she has left the surgery, you notice from her record that she is asthmatic. Which is the single most appropriate way to communicate to the patient not to take the medication? ★

A Ask the receptionist to make her a routine appointment for the next day

B Phone her and give her the appropriate advice

C Phone the local chemist and instruct them not to issue the prescription

D Phone the police and ask them to go to her house

E Write to her requesting her to make an urgent appointment

17. A 21-year-old single mother has a 2-month-old baby who is not sleeping and seems perpetually hungry. She is still breastfeeding, but thinks that she will have to change her baby to bottle-feeding. She wants some advice about this. Who is the single best person from the healthcare team to advise her? ★

A District nurse

B GP

C Health visitor

D Midwife

E Social worker

18. A 22-year-old woman has persistent headaches, nausea, and disturbed sleep. She appears very thin and her BMI is 16 kg/m². She tells you that this is her normal weight. Which single healthcare professional would it be most appropriate to refer her to? ★

A Counsellor

B Continue to see her yourself as a GP

C Dietitian

D Endocrinologist

E Psychiatrist

19. A 32-year-old woman is 33 weeks pregnant with her second child. She has come for a routine antenatal appointment. During her first pregnancy she had pre-eclampsia and required a hospital admission and early delivery. Today she is feeling tired and 'off colour.' Which single combination of clinical features would suggest that she could be suffering from pre-eclampsia requiring immediate hospital referral? ★

A Raised blood pressure alone

B Raised blood pressure and proteinuria

C Raised blood pressure, proteinuria, and headache

D Raised blood pressure, proteinuria, and peripheral oedema

E Raised blood pressure, proteinuria, and seizures

20. A 17-year-old man has had a sore throat, fever, malaise, and headache for 4 days. He has bilaterally enlarged tonsils with exudate, and cervical lymphadenopathy. Which single complication of his illness may be prevented by treatment with oral penicillin? ★

A Drug eruption

B Glomerulonephritis

C Mesenteric adenitis

D Otitis media

E Sinusitis

21. A 65-year-old woman with osteoarthritis affecting both knees is in need of some pain relief. However, she is unwilling to take anti-inflammatory drugs, as she says that they make her feel ill and pain-killers make her constipated. She asks whether complementary medicine could help her. Which single type of complementary medicine has the most evidence of efficacy? ★ ★

A Aromatherapy with oil of evening primrose.

B Glucosamine and chondroitin

C Homeopathy

D Modern acupuncture using trigger points

E Reflexology

22. A man has a chest infection. He is prescribed a course of amoxicillin for 1 week. He also wants a repeat prescription of his blood pressure medication. Under which single circumstance is he eligible to obtain the medications without paying prescription charges for them? ★

A He earns less than £25 000 per annum

B He has a partner and more than three children at home

C He has been unwell for more than 4 weeks

D He has diabetes

E He is aged over 50 years

23. A 35-year-old woman is 12 weeks pregnant. She has significant dysuria, urinary frequency, and offensive-smelling urine. A dip-stick test shows 3+ blood, 3+ leukocytes, and 2+ nitrites. Which single regime is the most appropriate treatment? ★ ★

A Amoxicillin for 7 days

B Encourage oral fluids and simple analgesia

C Nalidixic acid for 7 days

D Nitrofurantoin for 7 days

E Trimethoprim for 3 days

24. A 36-year-old woman attends the surgery for her 'pill check.' She has been on the combined hormonal contraceptive (CHC) Microgynon for 18 years, and wants to continue it as she has had no problems with it. She smokes 10 cigarettes a day. Her blood pressure is 140/88 mmHg and her BMI is 30 kg/m². Which is the single most appropriate management? ★ ★

A Explain that her blood pressure is too high for the CHC, and she needs to consider changing to an alternative method of contraception

B Explain that her BMI is too high for the CHC, and she needs to consider changing to an alternative method of contraception

C Explain that she has an increased risk of ovarian cancer on the CHC, and needs to consider changing to an alternative method of contraception

D Explain that smoking increases the risks associated with the CHC, and she needs to consider changing to an alternative method of contraception

E Give her a further prescription for Microgynon, and arrange a review in 6 months

25. A 50-year-old man seeks advice about his father, who has mild dementia and is living in a nursing home. The father is becoming increasingly unwell with a chest infection, and the son wants him to be admitted to hospital, but the father wishes to stay where he is. Which is the single best summary of the legal situation? ★ ★

A As the father has dementia, he is not competent and therefore the son can and should decide on his treatment

B The father is competent and can therefore decide on his own treatment, regardless of the son's opinion

C The father is not competent and therefore decisions about his care must be made by his doctor, based on the patient's best interests

D The father's competence should be assessed and, if he has capacity, he can accept or decline treatment himself regardless of the consequences

E The father's competence should be assessed, but his doctor may insist on admission, should his condition deteriorate, on the grounds of necessity

26. A 35-year-old woman with persistent irritable bowel syndrome asks to see a complementary therapist to help her with her symptoms. She understands that she may need to pay for this privately and that there may not be good evidence for the effectiveness of some complementary treatments, but she says that she is convinced that this is what she would like to do. Which is the single most appropriate action to take in response to her request? ★ ★

A Ask her to identify a practitioner whom she would like to see, and then provide a written referral if this is requested

B Decline to refer her on the grounds that this will avoid the need to pay private care fees

C Refer her directly to a colleague who runs a private complementary clinic

D Refer her to a gastroenterologist because she is more likely to achieve better symptom control with the help of a conventional specialist

E Refer her to a therapist selected from the Yellow Pages on the basis of geographical proximity to her home

27. A 65-year-old woman, who regularly attends with symptoms related to chronic depression, has some vague muscle ache and headache. She has been told before that her symptoms may well be related to her depression, but she requests further assessment. Which single aspect of her history is the most likely to point to a significant alternative diagnosis? ★ ★

A She has been experiencing pain in her hip when walking

B She has been experiencing some stinging pain on passing urine

C She has noticed a deterioration of her vision

D She has noticed some hearing loss in her left ear

E She has recently started taking herbal remedies for her depression

28. The local pharmacist has sent back a prescription that was written this morning. He says that a controlled drug has been prescribed wrongly—a patient with intractable chronic back pain has been given a prescription for morphine modified release (MST Continus®). Which single element must be on a prescription for a controlled drug? ★ ★

A The date must be written in words and figures

B The diagnosis must be specified

C The full name and address of the patient must be handwritten, not typed

D The prescriber's General Medical Council registration number must be given

E The total quantity to dispense must be expressed in words and figures

29. A medical student is sitting in on a GP surgery. One of the patients says that he would rather not have a student present. Which is the single most appropriate way of handling this? ★ ★ ★

A Before calling the patient in, ask the student to wait in another room

B Emphasize the importance of student teaching, hoping that the patient will reconsider

C Introduce the student and confirm that the patient would prefer the student to leave

D Rebook the patient for another surgery when you do not have students present

E Reschedule the patient to the end of surgery

30. A 62-year-old woman has had a unilateral painful rash highly suggestive of shingles for 36 hours. She asks if she could pass it on to her grandson, who is 7 days old. He lives in the same town and she last saw him yesterday. The baby's mother does not think she has ever had chickenpox. Which is the single most appropriate piece of advice to give to the grandmother? ★ ★ ★

A As the baby has been in contact with her, he should receive zoster immunoglobulin (ZIG) as soon as possible

B It is better to get chickenpox during childhood than later in life, and she need not worry about contact

C It is better to get shingles during childhood than later in life, and she need not worry about contact

D The baby could get chickenpox, and she should avoid seeing him until the blisters have crusted over

E The baby will be protected by maternal antibodies and will not be affected

31. A 40-year-old woman has heavy periods. Her periods have always been heavy but now they are getting worse and she wants to discuss possible treatments. She has no inter-menstrual or post-coital bleeding, and she is up to date with her cervical smears. She is otherwise well with no significant past medical history. She has two children and does not want any more. Her husband has had a vasectomy. Which is the single most appropriate management? ★ ★ ★

A Arrange blood tests, including a full blood count, a thyroid and hormone profile, and a pelvic ultrasound scan

B Conduct a pelvic examination and offer insertion of the Mirena coil

C Conduct a pelvic examination and offer the combined hormone contraceptive pill

D Refer her to gynaecology for consideration of endometrial ablation

E Refer her to gynaecology for consideration of hysterectomy

32. A 68-year-old man was watching television 10 days ago when his wife noticed that the right side of his face was drooping, his speech was slurred, and he could not move his right hand. This only lasted for 10 minutes, so he did not seek any medical help at the time. He has no other medical problems and is not on any medication. His blood pressure is 130/70 mmHg and examination is unremarkable. Which is the single most appropriate management? ★ ★ ★

A Admit him to hospital, as he has had a transient ischaemic attack (TIA) and is at high risk of progression to having a stroke

B Commence 75 mg aspirin and arrange blood tests, including cholesterol and glucose

C Commence 75 mg aspirin and refer him routinely to a medical clinic for further investigations

D Commence 300 mg aspirin and refer him to a TIA clinic to be seen within 24 hours

E Commence 300 mg aspirin and refer him to a TIA clinic to be seen within 1 week

Extended Matching Questions

Causes of chest pain

For each patient with acute chest pain, choose the *single* most likely diagnosis from the list of options below. Each option may be used once, more than once, or not at all. ★

A Bornholm's disease

B Costochondritis

C Dissecting aortic aneurysm

D Idiopathic chest pain

E Musculoskeletal chest pain

F Myocardial infarction

G Oesophageal spasm

H Pericarditis

I Pleurisy

J Pneumothorax

K Pulmonary embolus

L Shingles

1. A 63-year-old woman has had severe pain on the right side of her chest, over the right breast, for 2 days. The pain is constant and sharp, and is not affected by taking in a deep breath, coughing, or movement. She has no past medical history of note, is on no regular medication, and is a non-smoker. She is distressed by the pain, but is not sweaty or short of breath. Her pulse rate is 76 bpm and her blood pressure is 140/88 mmHg. She has some tenderness on the right side of her chest, with hyperaesthesia.

2. A 45-year-old man tore his right anterior cruciate ligament 5 days ago while skiing in Canada. It was repaired abroad and he has flown home. He has had sharp central chest pain for the past 8 hours, which is worse on taking a deep breath. He feels short of breath and is slightly sweaty. His respiratory rate is 25 breaths/minute, his blood pressure is 100/60 mmHg, his pulse rate is 100 bpm, and there is a pleural rub on the left side of his chest.

3. A 40-year-old woman has had chest pain for the last 4 days. The pain is worse on movement, coughing, or sneezing, and is slightly worse on taking in a deep breath. She feels very tired and has been unable to continue with her usual daily activity—she is a nurse at the local hospital and is married with three children. Her pulse rate is 68 bpm and regular, and her blood pressure is 120/82 mmHg. She has marked local tenderness to palpation on the left side, over her sternum, with no associated heat, erythema, or swelling.

4. A 55-year-old man has had central chest pain for 2 hours, radiating to his shoulders. The pain came on gradually over a few minutes while he was walking his dog, and is a tight pain or discomfort that feels like a pressure on his chest. It is not affected by position or coughing. He feels nauseated and sweaty, and is very anxious. He smokes 20 cigarettes a day. He looks clammy and is short of breath. His pulse rate is 88 bpm and his blood pressure is 110/60 mmHg. His heart sounds are normal and his chest sounds clear.

5. A 38-year-old woman has had a sharp, constant sternal pain for the last 24 hours, which came on suddenly. Prior to this, she had had a heavy head cold for 5 days. The pain radiates to the left shoulder and is worse if she is lying on her left side. Taking a deep breath, coughing, and swallowing also make it worse. The pain is relieved slightly by sitting forward. A scratchy rub can be heard over the left sternal border, which is louder when she leans forward.

Causes of dizziness

For each patient complaining of dizziness, choose the *single* most likely diagnosis from the list of options below. Each option may be used once, more than once, or not at all. ★

A Benign positional vertigo

B Cardiac arrhythmia

C Cerebellar disorder

D Cough syncope

E Hyperventilation

F Hypoglycaemia

G Ménière's syndrome

H Postural hypotension

I Pre-syncope

J Tumour

K Vertebrobasilar insufficiency

L Viral labyrinthitis

6. A 55-year-old man has type 1 diabetes and has had bouts of severe dizziness, lasting a few minutes each time, for 10 days. He has the sensation that his surroundings are spinning and he feels nauseated at the time. These episodes occur with changes in posture, and he has attacks up to ten times a day. They are not related to other activities, and he has been eating and checking his capillary blood glucose level as normal. He had a viral illness about 2 weeks ago. He has no nystagmus, Romberg's sign is negative, and his ENT examination is normal. He has a positive Hallpike test.

7. A 26-year-old man has type 1 diabetes. He had an episode of dizziness, which came on fairly rapidly over a period of a couple of minutes just before lunchtime at work. He had had an early start that day, but his capillary blood glucose level in the morning had been 7.0 mmol/L. He had a similar episode about 3 months earlier, also when he was at work. He appears clammy and sweaty, and generally unwell. His speech is slightly slurred.

8. A 21-year-old man had a sudden onset of vertigo, nausea, and vomiting 36 hours ago. He is unable to lift his head off the pillow because the room starts to spin if he does so. He has no loss of hearing, no tinnitus, and his ENT examination is normal. His pulse rate is 56 bpm and his blood pressure is 110/70 mmHg.

9. A 50-year-old woman has had dizziness and difficulty walking since she woke up 3 days ago. She has hypertension and is on bendroflumethiazide. She appears intoxicated, with a wide-based gait and slightly slurred speech. She is unable to walk in a straight line or to perform repetitive movements, and she has a rotary nystagmus in both eyes.

10. A 35-year-old woman has attacks of recurrent vertigo that started about 8 months ago. Attacks can come on at any time, and are associated with nausea and a feeling of fullness in the right ear. They last for up to 3 to 4 hours. She thinks that she may be becoming deaf on that side. Her grandmother had something similar. The tinnitus is 'driving her mad' and preventing her from sleeping.

Causes of fever

For each patient with fever, choose the *single* most likely diagnosis from the list of options below. Each option may be used once, more than once, or not at all. ★

A Appendicitis

B *Campylobacter* gastroenteritis

C Cholecystitis

D Hodgkin's lymphoma

E Malaria

F Meningococcal meningitis

G Menopausal flushing

H Pancreatitis

I Pneumonia

J Pyelonephritis

K Subacute bacterial endocarditis

L Tuberculosis

M Viral gastroenteritis

N Viral hepatitis

O Viral upper respiratory tract infection

11. A 27-year-old woman is generally unwell and feverish, with unusually dark urine. The next day she feels much worse and has diarrhoea and vomiting, with chills and sweating. Her temperature is 38.5°C. She last visited her GP 4 months ago for travel vaccinations prior to a holiday in Kenya.

12. A 3-year-old girl has had fever and vomiting for 2 days. She is not eating, is not sleeping well, and is crying more than usual. For the last day she has been very clingy and lethargic, and has not shown any interest in toys or games. She has a pink rash on her trunk that does not fade when pressed, and she is lethargic and floppy. Her temperature is 39°C.

13. A 40-year-old man who works as a chef has had diarrhoea, vomiting, and colicky abdominal pain for 3 days. The pain is centred around his umbilicus. The diarrhoea occurs up to fives times daily, and for the last day has been bloodstained. He mainly eats restaurant food, from the kitchen of the restaurant where he works.

14. A 19-year-old woman is in her first term at university. She has had a cough for the last 7 days, which is gradually getting worse. She has left-sided chest pain and is coughing up green sputum. She looks flushed, with a temperature of 39°C, a respiratory rate of 28 breaths/minute, and a pulse rate of 110 bpm. Her chest sounds clear on auscultation.

15. A 3-year-old girl has had a high temperature since the morning. She is off her food but is still drinking. She is clingy and her stools have been loose. She is snuffly and has a rough cough, with a barking quality. Her temperature is 40°C, and she is miserable but alert.

Causes of hypertension

For each patient scenario, choose the *single* most appropriate antihypertensive drug to prescribe from the list of options below. Each option may be used once, more than once, or not at all. ★ ★

A Amlodipine

B Atenolol

C Bendroflumethiazide

D Clonidine

E Doxazosin

F Furosemide

G Guanethidine

H Lisinopril

I Methyldopa

J No medications

K Propranolol

L Valsartan

16. A 36-year-old woman in the first trimester of pregnancy has had repeated blood pressure measurements of over 145/95 mmHg before and during pregnancy, but has no evidence of proteinuria or oedema.

17. A 65-year-old man with gout has a persistently raised blood pressure of 160/98 mmHg and has never been on blood pressure treatment.

18. A 45-year-old man has a raised blood pressure of 150/100 mmHg, and is not currently on any treatment.

19. A 34-year-old civil servant has a blood pressure of 135/80 mmHg. He is currently taking citalopram for panic disorder.

20. A 50-year-old woman is currently on enalapril to control her blood pressure. Her blood pressure is now 155/90 mmHg. She also has impaired glucose tolerance.

Causes of ENT problems

For each clinical situation, choose the *single* best management option from the list of options below. Each option may be used once, more than once, or not at all. ★ ★

A Combined antibiotic and steroid ear drops

B Nasal antihistamine spray

C Olive oil ear drops

D Oral aciclovir

E Oral antibiotics

F Oral antihistamine

G Reassure the patient and review them within 3 weeks

H Refer the patient for audiometry

I Refer the patient to the practice nurse for ear syringing

J Routine ENT referral

K Saline ear drops

L Urgent Emergency Department referral

M Urgent ENT referral

21. A 35-year-old man has noticed a decline in his hearing over the last few months. He has bilateral impacted wax in his ear canals.

22. A 25-year-old swimmer has had a painful left ear for 2 days. The left ear canal is red and swollen, and there is some yellow crusting. The tympanic membrane can be seen and is intact.

23. A 35-year-old woman has hurt her right ear today while cleaning it with a cotton bud. There is swelling of the ear canal, and the tympanic membrane is not visible due to the swelling and the presence of blood.

24. A 4-year-old boy is brought in by his mother who thinks that his hearing is reduced. He is interacting normally with his family and is generally well.

25. A 55-year-old man has increasing pain and hearing loss in his left ear. There are crusting vesicles in the ear canal.

ANSWERS

Single Best Answers

1. C ★

BMI is calculated as weight in kilograms divided by height in metres squared (kg/m^2). It is a measure of weight for height and does not represent body fat or other ratios.

2. A ★   OHCS 9th edn → p. 770

Retention of urine and faeces should raise suspicions of cauda equina syndrome (compression of the cauda equina in the spinal canal). Pain and inability to perform a straight leg raise can be caused by muscular back injury or sciatica, and ankle jerks are usually brisk in cord compression.

3. C ★

All competent patients have a right to confidentiality, and you should not break this unless the patient specifically gives consent for you to share the information. However, if the mother wants to express her concerns about her daughter, it is acceptable to listen to these without revealing any information.

→ www.gmc-uk.org/guidance/current/library/confidentiality.asp

4. E ★

There are several risk factors for stroke, some of which can be modified and some of which cannot. Hypertension is considered to be the most important risk factor for stroke, with well-documented relationships between blood pressure and the occurrence of stroke. There is also good evidence that treating hypertension reduces the risk of stroke.

5. C ★   OHCS 9th edn → p. 532

An approach that is patient-centred and which identifies, acknowledges, and respects the patient's decisions and feelings ensures a better long-term result. It is important to realize that all patients have different life factors that may influence their decision making. Respecting these is vital for building a lasting relationship.

6. D ★

All of these are possible risk factors for poor sleep, apart from moderate cigarette smoking. However, the suggestion of low mood and possible depression is an important presenting symptom that needs to be followed up.

7. E ★   OHCS 9th edn → p. 272

HPV can cause cervical abnormalities that may progress to become cancer. There are hundreds of HPVs, of which types 16 and 18 cause 70% of HPV-related cervical cancers. HPV types 6 and 11 are associated with genital warts. In the UK, two vaccines are currently used. Cervarix immunizes against types 16 and 18, and Gardasil immunizes against types 6, 11, 16, and 18. The current programme schedule involves three doses given at 0, 1–2, and 6 months. The Department of Health recommends that any women under the age of 18 years with unknown or incomplete immunization status should complete the course. Those from overseas who are not protected should be offered protection.

Department of Health. *Immunisation Against Infectious Disease ('the Green Book')*:

→ www.dh.gov.uk/en/Publichealth/Healthprotection/Immunisation/
Greenbook/index.htm

8. D ★

A common-sense approach to difficult situations such as this that respects the main principles of patient autonomy, beneficence, and non-maleficence is needed here. GPs may have to help patients to interpret health information, especially now that they have access to so much more information via the Internet.

9. E ★   OHCS 9th edn → p. 530

Type 2 diabetes is greatly increased in overweight people and is a major cause of morbidity. A healthy body mass index (BMI) is in the range of 20–25 kg/m^2. If this woman lost 20 kg, her weight would be 65 kg. Her BMI would therefore be $65/1.6^2$, which is 25.4 kg/m^2. This is a much healthier BMI and an achievable range to aim for.

→ www.nice.org.uk/nicemedia/pdf/word/CG43NICEGuideline.doc

10. D ★

A possible diagnosis is malaria, which would be suspected if the patient had travelled to a region where malaria is prevalent.

11. D ★

Influenza vaccine is prepared each year from viruses of the three strains that are thought most likely to cause flu that winter. It is about 70% effective, and protection lasts for 1 year. Pneumococcal vaccine only needs to be given once. Both are recommended for high-risk groups of patients, including individuals with diabetes.

→ www.dh.gov.uk/en/Publichealth/Immunisation/Greenbook/index.htm

12. **E** ★

Although all patients are entitled to appropriate treatment, you should not place other patients or practice staff at risk of harm. This patient has the same right to treatment as do others, but you should not disadvantage other patients by seeing him first simply because he is demanding. It may be necessary to call the police, but you may well be able to advise and treat him without difficulty, and you should endeavour to do this before taking more drastic action.

13. **D** ★

The occupational therapist's role is to assess patients with regard to their activities of daily living, and to advise on how to make these activities achievable.

14. **B** ★

Glandular fever or infectious mononucleosis, caused by Epstein–Barr virus, can cause splenomegaly. A rare but serious complication is splenic rupture, the risk of which is increased by contact sports and trauma to the area. The splenomegaly usually lasts for 6 to 8 weeks.

15. **D** ★   OHCS 9th edn → p. 301

The Pill can increase the risk of ischaemic stroke. Women who have a history of migraine should stop the Pill immediately if they develop aura and worsening headache, and should have an ischaemic event excluded if these symptoms persist. The progestogen-only pill is a safe alternative, as it contains no oestrogen, which is the component that leads to the increased risk.

→ www.bnf.org/bnf (see Section 7.3.1; requires registration)

→ www.fsrh.org/pdfs/CEUGuidanceCombinedHormonalContraception. pdf

16. **B** ★

NSAIDs may cause worsening of asthma, although this is not always the case. However, the patient should be warned about the risk and advised not to take the medication. The most effective way to ensure that this is done is to speak to her yourself. A further appointment can be offered to discuss alternative treatments later.

17. **C** ★   OHCS 9th edn → p. 474

The health visitor is a qualified nurse with a health visiting qualification (which includes public health nursing and health promotion). She takes over home visiting of new mothers from the midwife when the baby is 10 days old.

18. E ★   OHCS 9th edn → p. 348

There is a high probability that this woman has anorexia nervosa, and with a persistently low BMI below 17 kg/m², she needs to be assessed and managed by a psychiatrist with a particular interest in eating disorders. You may of course continue to see her as a GP, but she needs specialist help to direct her treatment.

19. C ★   OHCS 9th edn → p. 48

Pre-eclampsia is defined as hypertension plus proteinuria, with or without peripheral oedema. However, the presence of symptoms such as headache makes hospital referral important here. The presence of seizures would make the diagnosis eclampsia, rather than pre-eclampsia.

20. B ★

Although there is no clear evidence to support the use of antibiotics to reduce the incidence of post-streptococcal glomerulonephritis, antibiotics are often given in primary care for this reason.

21. B ★ ★

Many patients seek complementary therapies, so it is useful to have some idea of the more common ones and those for which there is an evidence base. Glucosamine may be helpful in large-joint arthritis.

→ http://jama.ama-assn.org/cgi/content/abstract/283/11/1469

→ www.nice.org.uk/nicemedia/live/11926/39554/39554.pdf

22. D ★

This patient would qualify for free prescriptions if he was aged over 60 years, and if he had a low income and less than £16 000 in savings or investments, or if he had one of a number of chronic diseases. Help is based on a comparison between an individual's weekly income and assessed requirements at the time when the claim is made (or the date on which the charge was paid if a refund is claimed).

→ www.nhsbsa.nhs.uk/HealthCosts/Documents/HealthCosts/HC11.pdf

23. D ★ ★

This patient clearly has a significant urinary tract infection and needs antibiotic treatment. Trimethoprim and nalidixic acid are contraindicated in the first trimester of pregnancy, and amoxicillin, although safe, is likely to be ineffective due to widespread resistance. Nitrofurantoin is safe in early pregnancy but is best avoided near term, because of the possible risk of haemolytic anaemia in newborn babies.

24. D ★★

When re-prescribing 'the Pill', blood pressure and BMI should be recorded, as well as smoking history and whether the patient is having any problems. A smoking history is important because both smoking and the oral CHC can increase the risk of venous thromboembolism. The cut-off age for prescribing the Pill in a smoker is 35 years. There is no evidence that a lower-strength pill decreases this risk. Although this woman's BMI is raised and she is obese, the cut-off BMI for prescribing the pill is 35 kg/m^2. CHC use may be associated with a small increase in the risk of cervical cancer, which is related to duration of use, and a small increased risk of breast cancer, which will reduce with time after stopping, but a reduced risk of ovarian and endometrial cancer that continues for several decades after stopping. A persistently raised blood pressure over 160/95 mmHg would mean that this patient should stop the pill and consider an alternative, which could include a progesterone-only pill, depot or implant, or an IUD or IUS.

→ www.fsrh.org/pdfs/CEUGuidanceCombinedHormonalContraception.pdf

25. D ★★ OHCS 9th edn → p. 402

The patient may have capacity, but it needs to be assessed. If he is competent, he can refuse or accept any treatment that is offered. However, he cannot insist on treatment that is not considered appropriate by his doctor. This legal situation is covered by different Acts in England and Wales, and in Scotland.

26. A ★★

Provided that you are happy that the patient is not at risk of harm, it is appropriate to facilitate a referral to a complementary therapist if they request it. However, because this is a private referral, you need to ensure that it is done professionally, that the patient has as much choice as possible, and that there is no suggestion that you have a personal interest in the referral.

27. C ★★

A wide variety of symptoms can occur in depression. However, it is important always to revisit the diagnosis and to assess every presentation fully. In an elderly woman with headaches and myalgia, loss of vision may occur in giant-cell arteritis, and prompt treatment can save sight.

28. E ★★

Prescriptions for controlled drugs must be indelible and include:

- the name and address of the patient
- the form and strength of the preparation
- the total quantity in both words and figures of the preparation, or the number in both words and figures of dosage units, to be supplied
- the dose to be given
- the prescriber's name, signature, and address
- the date of the prescription.

Pharmacists cannot dispense unless the prescription is filled in correctly.

→ www.bnf.org/bnf/bnf/57/29424.htm (requires registration)

29. A ★★★

When asking a patient whether they will allow a student to be present, you should have an appropriate mechanism to ensure that this does not pressurize the patient, embarrass either them or the student, or disadvantage the patient in any way.

30. A ★★★   OHCS 9th edn→ p. 144

Neonates with significant exposure to chickenpox or shingles should receive ZIG as soon as possible. The fact that the mother has probably never had chickenpox means that she has no varicella antibodies to pass across the placenta, and the baby therefore has no protection.

31. B ★★★★

The National Institute for Health and Clinical Excellence (NICE) has provided guidelines on the management of heavy periods. These suggest that in simple heavy menstrual bleeding the only investigation required is a full blood count to rule out anaemia. A pelvic examination is only required if a structural or histological abnormality is suspected, or an intrauterine device is being considered. The first-line recommended treatment is a Mirena coil, with treatments such as non-steroidal anti-inflammatory drugs, tranexamic acid, and combined hormone contraceptives being second-line treatment. Surgical management is considered if pharmaceutical treatments have failed, and/or there is a severe impact on the woman's quality of life, after full discussion of the risks.

→ www.fsrh.org/pdfs/archive/LNG-IUS0404.pdf

→ www.nice.org.uk/nicemedia/live/11002/30401/30401.pdf

32. E ★ ★ ★ ★

A transient ischaemic attack (TIA) is defined as stroke symptoms and signs that resolve within 24 hours. Patients who present with a TIA need to be assessed to determine whether they are at high or low risk using the validated ABCD (Age, Blood pressure, Clinical features, Duration of symptoms and Diabetes) tool. A patient with an ABCD score higher than 4 is at high risk and should have specialist assessment and investigations, such as cholesterol and carotid Dopplers, within 24 hours. Patients with a score of less than 4 or who present more than 1 week after the event should have specialist assessment and investigation within 1 week. This man has a score of 3, and is therefore at low risk. All patients should be started on 300 mg of aspirin, unless this is contraindicated.

→ www.nice.org.uk/nicemedia/live/12018/41331/41331.pdf

Extended Matching Questions

1. L ★

Shingles is a reactivation of latent chickenpox, and the pain of shingles usually pre-dates the vesicular rash by 2 to 3 days. It can be confused with other conditions, as the skin looks clear in the early stages and the pain can be very severe. Shingles develops from the dorsal root ganglion within which it has been latent, and therefore never crosses the midline. It also follows the line of the dermatome, sometimes also within an adjacent dermatome.

2. K ★

A pulmonary embolus should be suspected in any patient who presents with chest pain and shortness of breath following an operation, especially if they are not anticoagulated. In this case, the long-haul flight home is an additional risk factor. Other risk factors include smoking, the oral contraceptive pill, pregnancy or puerperium, malignancy, and a past history of deep vein thrombosis or pulmonary embolism. Many of the signs of pulmonary embolism are also common in patients without a pulmonary embolus, which is why the history is so important to raise suspicion of the diagnosis. This patient would need urgent referral to hospital.

3. B ★

Chest wall-related causes are among the commonest reasons for chest pain seen by GPs. Sometimes the patient may describe repetitive movements or unaccustomed activity that might account for the development of the pain. Costochondritis is one of the more common presentations of musculoskeletal chest pain. It is a diffuse pain syndrome, in which multiple areas of tenderness are found that reproduce the described pain. The upper costal cartilages at the costochondral or costosternal junctions are most frequently involved.

Plate 1.1

Plate 1.2

Plate 2.1

Infants receiving phototherapy must have a minimum
of BD bilirubin estimations

Plate 2.2

Plate 2.3

Plate 2.4

Plate 2.5

Plate 2.6

Plate 2.7

Plate 4.1

Plate 4.2

Plate 4.3

Plate 4.4

Plate 4.5

Plate 4.6

Plate 6.1

Plate 7.1

Plate 7.2

Plate 7.3

Plate 7.4

Plate 7.5

Plate 7.6

Plate 7.7

Plate 7.8

Plate 7.9

Plate 7.10

Plate 7.11

Plate 7.12

Plate 7.13

Plate 7.14

Plate 7.15

Plate 7.16

Plate 7.17

Plate 7.18a

Plate 7.18b

Plate 7.19

Plate 7.20

Plate 7.21

Plate 7.22

Plate 7.23

Plate 7.24

Plate 7.25

Plate 7.26

Plate 7.27

Plate 7.28

Plate 7.29

Plate 7.30

Plate 7.31

Plate 7.32

Plate 7.33

Plate 7.34

Plate 7.35

Plate 7.36

Plate 7.37

Plate 7.38

Plate 7.39

Plate 7.40

Plate 7.41

Plate 7.42

Plate 7.43

Plate 7.44

Plate 7.45

Plate 7.46

Plate 7.47

Plate 7.48

Plate 7.49

Plate 7.50

Plate 7.51

Plate 7.52

Plate 7.53

Plate 7.54

Plate 7.55

Plate 7.56

Plate 7.57

Plate 7.58

Plate 7.59

Plate 8.1

Plate 9.1

Plate 9.2

Plate 9.3

Plate 9.4

Plate 9.5

Plate 9.6

Plate 10.1

4. F ★

This patient is assumed to be having a MI unless proven otherwise. It is difficult to tell the difference between acute MI and unstable angina in general practice, but the treatment is similar. An ECG may look normal at this stage. This patient requires urgent admission to hospital for consideration of thrombolysis or angioplasty, as this needs to be given as soon as possible. He should also be given aspirin (300 mg) immediately if there is no contraindication, and he may need IV diamorphine and an anti-emetic. If his systolic blood pressure is higher than 90 mmHg and his pulse rate is higher than 100 bpm, he should also be given sublingual glyceryl trinitrate to act as a coronary vasodilator.

5. H ★

Initial evaluation should consider disorders that are known to involve the pericardium, such as uraemia, recent myocardial infarction, and previous cardiac surgery. Other causes include infection (e.g. Coxsackie virus, tuberculosis), malignancy, trauma, connective tissue disease, and hypothyroidism. The examination should pay particular attention to auscultation for a pericardial friction rub and the signs associated with tamponade. The patient should be assessed that day by a cardiologist, and if the pain is thought to be due to an uncomplicated viral pericarditis, she can be treated as an outpatient with non-steroidal anti-inflammatory drugs to control the pain and inflammation.

6. A ★

Benign positional vertigo lasts for only a few seconds or minutes, and occurs with sudden changes of position. It may be caused by otoliths in the labyrinth of the inner ear, and is common after head injury or viral illness, and increases in diabetes. Diagnosis is made on the basis of history and a positive Hallpike test. Sit the patient up with their legs extended and rotate the head 45°. Then ask them to lie down quickly with the head extended. After about 10 seconds, rotational nystagmus will occur with the fast phase towards the affected ear. The condition may be self-limiting, and can be treated successfully in the GP surgery by using the Epley manoeuvre.

→ www.cks.nhs.uk/benign_paroxysmal_positional_vertigo#-471817

7. F ★

These are the symptoms and signs of hypoglycaemia. On this particular day the patient had to start work early, and had not had time to eat his usual mid-morning snack. This resulted in a hypoglycaemic attack. The diagnosis can be made quickly by checking his capillary blood glucose level.

8. L ★

Viral labyrinthitis usually follows a viral respiratory tract infection. It can be treated symptomatically with labyrinthine sedatives, such as cyclizine or prochlorperazine. It usually resolves within 2 to 3 weeks. If the symptoms persist for more than 6 weeks, the patient should be referred to an ENT specialist.

9. C ★

This patient is demonstrating signs of cerebellar dysfunction. The cause of this is not known from this history and examination, and the patient will need to be referred urgently for further tests, including a CT scan of the brain. The most likely diagnosis is cerebellar stroke, but this patient could also have a cerebellar tumour or multiple sclerosis, among other possible diagnoses.

10. G ★

This is a complex of symptoms that include clustering of attacks of vertigo and nausea, tinnitus, a sense of fullness in the ear, and sensorineural deafness, which may be progressive. All cases should be referred for confirmation of the diagnosis. In this case, the unilateral nature of the patient's symptoms would mean that an acoustic neuroma should be excluded.

> *General feedback on 6–10:* OHCS 9th edn → pp. 554–555
>
> 'Dizziness' is a non-specific term used by patients to describe symptoms, so it is vital to obtain as precise a description of the sensation as possible in order to establish the cause. The distribution of causes varies with age. Patients often experience vertigo as an illusion of motion; some interpret this as self-motion, others as motion of the environment. All vertigo is made worse by moving the head. This is a very useful symptom for distinguishing vertigo from other forms of dizziness. The presence of additional neurological signs strongly suggests the presence of a central vestibular lesion. Symptoms such as staggering or ataxic gait, vomiting, headache, double vision, visual loss, slurred speech, numbness of the face or body, weakness, clumsiness, or incoordination should be reviewed with the patient. Positional changes in symptoms, orthostatic blood pressure and pulse changes, observation of gait, and detection of nystagmus are helpful on physical examination.

11. E ★

Malaria should be excluded first, by doing a full blood count and thin and thick films to look for malaria parasites, and a rapid antigen test if this is available locally. If the patient is clinically very unwell, she needs urgent admission. Malaria is a notifiable disease, and 2000 cases per year are notified in the UK. *Plasmodium falciparum* malaria can be fatal within less than 24 hours, especially if it occurs in very young children.

→ www.hpa.org.uk/Topics/InfectiousDiseases/InfectionsAZ/Malaria/ GeneralInformation/mala10Background/

12. **F** ★

A non-blanching rash in a floppy lethargic child is highly suggestive of meningococcal sepsis. The GP should call 999 and get the patient to hospital quickly, and he or she should also give her a stat IM bolus of benzylpenicillin. For a 3-year-old child this should be 600 mg (1.2 g for an adult or for a child over 10 years of age, and 300 mg for an infant under 1 year).

13. **B** ★

The GP should send off a stool sample for analysis. In the mean time, they should ask the chef not to go into work until a clear stool sample has been obtained. If the stool sample is positive for *Campylobacter*, the GP should notify the public health service and treat the patient with ciprofloxacin.

→ www.hpa.org.uk/Topics/InfectiousDiseases/InfectionsAZ/Campylo
bacter/GeneralInformation/campyCampylobacterFAQs/

14. **I** ★

The clinical findings may not show a left-sided consolidation—it may be necessary to make the decision based on the patient's overall clinical condition. The British Thoracic Society has produced guidelines for assessing the severity of community-acquired pneumonia. As this woman is tachycardic and tachypnoeic, she may require admission for treatment with intravenous antibiotics.

→ www.brit-thoracic.org.uk/Portals/0/Clinical%20Information/
Pneumonia/Guidelines/MACAPrevisedApr04.pdf

15. **O** ★

This patient probably has a mild form of croup, which is a viral infection. She needs fluids and paracetamol, and the GP should give the parents details of the symptoms that they should look out for, or guidelines on when to call the doctor again if she is not getting better (e.g. if she develops a non-blanching rash, if she stops drinking, or if her temperature is not controlled by paracetamol).

→ www.nice.org.uk/nicemedia/pdf/CG47NICEGuideline.pdf

16. **I** ★★

17. **A** ★★

18. **H** ★★

19. **J** ★★

20. A ★★

> *General feedback on 16–20:* In England and Wales, the National Institute for Health and Clinical Excellence (NICE) has produced guidelines on the treatment of hypertension. These cover lifestyle factors that should be considered and modified first, and assessment of other risk factors, such as age and ethnicity. The choice of treatment (or no treatment) depends on these factors. In Scotland, the Scottish Intercollegiate Guidelines Network (SIGN) has produced similar guidelines. Concurrent medical conditions may determine which treatment should be given. For example, diuretics can be harmful in gout. In pregnancy, methyldopa is usually the drug of choice, but it is not used routinely in other situations.
>
> → www.nice.org.uk/nicemedia/live/13561/56008/56008.pdf
> → www.sign.ac.uk/guidelines/fulltext/49/section5.html
> → http://bnf.org/bnf/bnf/current/2534.htm (registration required)

21. C ★★

Olive oil drops help the ear to clean itself, and are effective for the treatment of excess wax that is causing symptoms. Syringing can lead to an increased risk of ear infections and perforations, so is not a first-line treatment.

22. A ★★

This is otitis externa—that is, infection of the external auditory meatus. Combined drops are the most effective treatment for this disorder.

23. M ★★

Cotton buds can damage the ear, can cause trauma and infection, and can actually push wax further down and cause it to become impacted. In this case, there seems to be an acute injury and possibly damage to the tympanic membrane, which might need intervention.

24. H ★★

As children cannot tell you whether their hearing is reduced, parental concern should always be taken seriously. Audiometry will reveal whether the boy does have impaired hearing, which could be due to a number of causes, of which the commonest is fluid in the middle ear.

25. D ★★

Herpes zoster (shingles) in the ear causes pain and the development of vesicles. It can progress to hearing loss, vertigo, and facial palsy. As it is viral, it can be treated with aciclovir.

> *General feedback on 21–25:* OHCS 9th edn → pp. 538, 540, 542

ENT

Philippa Tostevin

Ear, nose, and throat surgery is a fascinating specialty, which is involved in the diagnosis and management of a vast range of diseases presenting from birth through all ages. The pathologies covered range from congenital airway obstruction in the neonate to head and neck malignancies in elderly patients. Systemic diseases can also manifest for the first time in the ENT area. The creation of a surgical airway in the form of a tracheostomy can be life-saving, but some ENT surgery is performed to improve quality of life, so it is particularly important to understand the indications for surgical interventions. In contrast to other surgical specialties, many of the patients who are seen in the outpatient setting do not need surgery, and medical management is required.

For those interested in ENT surgery as a career, there are different areas within this diverse field that can be followed to a specialist level. These include rhinology, otology, and neuro-otology, in addition to the specialist areas of paediatric ENT, head and neck cancer surgery, voice, and facial plastic surgery.

A thorough knowledge and understanding of the diagnosis and management of common ENT conditions is vital for those who wish to work in general practice, paediatrics, or emergency medicine. ENT conditions in children represent a very large proportion of the workload in any general practice setting. Various foreign bodies can be swallowed, inhaled, or inserted into the nose or ear, so an understanding of how and when these need to be removed is essential for any junior doctor working in the Emergency Department.

In this chapter, the questions are based on the important knowledge that needs to be accrued as an undergraduate, as many readers may not have the opportunity to work as a junior doctor in an ENT team before treating ENT patients in the Emergency Department or in a general practice setting.

QUESTIONS

Single Best Answers

1. A 78-year-old man has sudden onset of hoarse voice. He has a weak cough and he coughs when eating. He has been a smoker since the age of 18 years. He has a right-sided vocal cord palsy. Which is the single most likely anatomical site for his primary malignancy? ★

A Bronchus

B Larynx

C Oesophagus

D Oral cavity

E Parotid

2. A 32-year-old lorry driver has had a painless, discharging left ear for 10 years. His Weber test lateralizes to the left and his Rinne test is negative on the left and positive on the right. The external auditory meatus is filled with mucopurulent debris. Which is the single most likely diagnosis? ★

A Chronic otitis externa

B Chronic secretory otitis media

C Chronic suppurative otitis media

D Malignant otitis externa

E Middle ear effusion

3. A 66-year-old man has a unilateral, non-pulsatile tinnitus that is keeping him awake at night. His pure-tone audiogram shows asymmetrical sensorineural hearing loss. Which single benign tumour may be responsible for these findings? ★

A Astrocytoma

B Glioma

C Meningioma

D Pleomorphic adenoma

E Vestibular schwannoma

4. A 76-year-old woman has right-sided otalgia and vertigo. Her Rinne test is positive in both ears and her Weber test lateralizes to the left ear. There are vesicles present on the superior aspect of her right pinna and drooping of her face on the right side. Which single virus is most likely to have caused this clinical presentation? ★

A Adenovirus

B Cytomegalovirus

C Epstein–Barr virus

D Herpes simplex virus

E Varicella zoster virus

5. A 23-year-old man has a 2 cm ulcer in his oral cavity. He has lost 3 kg in weight over the last 3 months. The edge of the ulcer is biopsied and the histopathology result shows non-caseating granulomata. Which is the single most likely diagnosis? ★

A Actinomycosis

B Crohn's disease

C Tuberculosis

D Ulcerative colitis

E Vitamin B$_{12}$ deficiency

6. A 23-year-old woman has had a fall at the gym. She now has a transient sensation of movement when she turns her head to the right. There is no hearing loss or tinnitus. Which is the single most likely diagnosis? ★

A Benign paroxysmal positional vertigo

B Labyrinthitis

C Ménière's disease

D Temporal bone fracture

E Vestibular neuronitis

7. A 17-year-old man has sudden-onset hearing loss after standing near an exploding firework. He has a central perforation of the tympanic membrane and a conductive hearing loss. Which is the single most appropriate acute management? ★

A Emergency myringoplasty

B Grommet insertion

C Intravenous antibiotics

D Keep the ear dry and review

E Topical antibiotic and steroid drops

8. A 26-year-old man has had a foul-smelling, painless otorrhoea and a conductive hearing loss for 3 years. There is moist white debris in the attic of the right tympanic membrane. Which is the single most appropriate next intervention? ★

A Daily suction toilet

B Intravenous antibiotics

C Mastoid exploration

D Myringoplasty

E Ventilation tube insertion

9. A 63-year-old man has otalgia and a hard, craggy mass on the right tonsil. He has been a smoker for the last 40 years. Which is the single most likely histological type of tumour? ★

A Adenocarcinoma

B Lymphoma

C Rhabdomyosarcoma

D Small-cell carcinoma

E Squamous cell carcinoma

10. A 75-year-old woman has had a hoarse voice, lethargy, and weight gain for 8 weeks. On examination, her vocal cords appear thickened. Which single blood test is most likely to be helpful in making a diagnosis? ★

A Full blood count

B Liver function test

C Serum calcium level

D Thyroid function test

E Urea and electrolytes

11. A 3-year-old girl is snoring so loudly that she is keeping the family awake. She has never had tonsillitis, but an overnight sleep study has shown desaturations to 80% in room air when she is asleep. The oropharyngeal examination is shown in Plate 6.1 (see Colour Plate section). Which is the single most appropriate management? ★

A Adenotonsillectomy

B Continuous home oxygen at night

C Continuous positive airway pressure (CPAP) via a face mask at night

D Palatal stiffening procedure

E Tonsillectomy

12. A 63-year-old diabetic man has an intensely itchy and painful right ear. Spores are seen in the external auditory meatus, which are cleared with microsuction. Which is the single most appropriate management? ★

A Aluminium acetate ear drops

B Glycerine and ichthammol

C Intravenous voriconazole

D Oral ketoconazole

E Topical clotrimazole

13. A 2-year-old boy has a temperature of 39°C and purulent otorrhoea. His pinna is laterally and inferiorly displaced, but the post-auricular sulcus is maintained. Which is the single most appropriate first-line emergency management? ★

A Admit the patient for analgesia and observation

B Admit the patient for intravenous antibiotics

C Emergency grommet insertion

D Give antibiotic ear drops

E Give oral antibiotics

14. A 70-year-old man has had an intermittently discharging ear for 5 years. He has come for review. Which single new clinical finding would indicate that he may have developed a malignancy? ★

A Black spores in the external auditory meatus

B Circumferential oedema of the external auditory meatus

C Offensive-smelling discharge

D Purulent discharge

E Sanguineous discharge

15. A 20-year-old man has chronic facial pain and rhinorrhoea. He has had multiple courses of antibiotics, with little improvement in his symptoms. A coronal CT scan of his paranasal sinuses shows a round opacity with mixed density within the right maxillary sinus. Which is the single most likely explanation for these findings? ★ ★

A Allergic polyp

B Angiofibroma

C Antrochoanal polyp

D Fungal ball

E Foreign body within the sinus

16. A 4-year-old boy with Down's syndrome has a proven middle-ear effusion bilaterally that has been present for 6 months. His pure-tone hearing thresholds are 40 dB bilaterally. Which is the single most appropriate management? ★ ★

A Adenoidectomy

B Bilateral mastoidectomy

C Bilateral ventilation tube insertion

D Cochlea implantation

E Watch and wait for 3 months

17. A 68-year-old woman has otalgia and dysphagia. She has angular cheilitis and pale conjunctivae. Her oropharyngeal examination is normal. In which single anatomical site is this patient likely to have a tumour? ★ ★

A Lower oesophagus

B Nasopharynx

C Post-cricoid

D Thyroid

E Tonsil

18. A 47-year-old woman has pulsatile tinnitus in her right ear. Her hearing is normal. There is a red lesion visible on the promontory in the middle ear behind the tympanic membrane. Which is the single most likely diagnosis? ★ ★

A Arteriovenous malformation

B Carotid body tumour

C Glomus tumour

D Middle-ear polyp

E Otosclerosis

19. A 72-year-old woman with rheumatoid arthritis has hoarseness of her voice. There is a left vocal cord palsy. Which single joint is likely to be involved? ★ ★

A Atlanto-occipital

B Cricoarytenoid

C Cricothyroid

D Costochondral

E Sternoclavicular

20. A 32-year-old woman is having intermittent episodes of vertigo. Each episode lasts for up to 12 hours, with associated tinnitus and hearing loss. Which single medication may be of help in reducing the frequency of her vertiginous episodes? ★ ★

A Amitriptyline

B Betahistine

C Cyclizine

D Paroxetine

E Prochlorperazine

21. A 2-year-old girl had an episode of acute otitis media 3 weeks ago. She now has no pain or temperature, but has a residual hearing loss. A type B tympanometry trace is found with a normal canal volume measurement. Which is the single most likely explanation for this result? ★ ★

A Cholesteatoma

B Chronic suppurative otitis media

C Perforation of the tympanic membrane

D Persistent acute otitis media

E Serous middle-ear effusion

22. A 5-year-old boy has a submandibular lump. It is non-tender with a light purplish discolouration of the overlying skin. He is apyrexial and otherwise well. His GP has tried several courses of anti-biotics, but the lump has continued to grow. Which is the single most likely diagnosis? ★ ★

A Atypical mycobacterial infection

B Brucellosis

C Infectious mononucleosis

D Lymphoma

E Toxoplasmosis

23. A 76-year-old man has acute disabling vertigo with nausea and vomiting. He has no tinnitus, and normal hearing. He has an intention tremor. Which single test would be most helpful in establishing a diagnosis? ★ ★

A Audiogram

B Brainstem-evoked response testing

C Caloric testing

D CT scan of brain

E Otoacoustic emissions

24. A 47-year-old opera singer presented to the ENT clinic with loss of vocal range. Nasendoscopic examination revealed bilateral vocal cord nodules. Which single initial treatment option should be offered to this patient? ★ ★

A Laser ablation of the nodule

B Microdebridement of the nodule

C Propranolol

D Sharp dissection of the nodule

E Voice therapy

25. A 3-year-old child presents with periorbital oedema and chemosis. Her right eye is proptosed and the eye movement is restricted. Which is the single most appropriate imaging technique to reveal any subperiosteal abscess formation in the orbit? ★ ★ ★

A CT angiogram

B CT scan

C MRI scan

D Ultrasound scan

E Sinus X-ray

26. A 2-year-old boy was playing with a small plastic toy and then began coughing for 2 minutes. His mother called 999. He is now completely well and eating and drinking normally, but the toy is nowhere to be found. Which is the single most appropriate management? ★ ★ ★

A CT scan of the chest

B Microlaryngoscopy and bronchoscopy

C Nasendoscopy in the Emergency Department

D Flexible oesophagogastroduodenoscopy

E Rigid oesophagoscopy

27. A 23-year-old woman has fallen from a tree on to her face. She has a nasal fracture and clear rhinorrhoea. The nasal discharge is positive for glucose. Which single test would you ask for to confirm the nature of the nasal fluid? ★ ★ ★

A Albumin

B β-Galactosidase

C β-2 Transferrin

D Ferritin

E Myoglobin

28. A 16-year-old boy sustains a nasal fracture during a game of football. He feels that his nose is obstructed. Both nasal bones are in the midline and both nasal airways are obscured by red swollen mucosa, which is soft when palpated. Which is the single most appropriate first step in management? ★ ★ ★

A Incision and drainage

B Manipulation of the nasal fracture

C Oral antibiotics and review

D Rhinoplasty

E Septoplasty

29. At 7pm, a 3-year-old girl is brought to the Emergency Department having pushed a lithium battery up her nose earlier in the afternoon. It cannot be removed in the department. Which is the single most appropriate time to list her for removal of the battery under general anaesthetic? ★ ★ ★

A After a course of steroids to decrease the inflammation

B After waiting a few days for the inflammation to subside

C On the next available elective list

D This evening, as soon as possible

E Tomorrow morning

30. Following his laryngectomy operation, a 74-year-old man has his speech restored using a valve in a tracheo-oesophageal fistula. The speech therapist wishes to explain to him the mechanism whereby he is able to communicate again. Which is the single best description of the mechanism for his post-laryngectomy speech restoration? ★ ★ ★ ★

A A hand-held resonating device is used in conjunction with the valve to create speech

B A fenestrated tracheostomy tube is fitted to enable speech restoration

C Air from the lungs is diverted through the valve and up to the pharynx, which vibrates to create sound

D Air from the lungs is diverted through the valve, which vibrates to create sound

E Air is taken into the oesophagus, and this causes the valve to vibrate

31. A 37-year-old man has an epistaxis that has not been controlled with 24 hours of nasal packing and bed rest. His blood pressure is 120/72 mmHg. A decision to perform arterial ligation is made. Which single artery is most commonly ligated first in this situation? ★ ★ ★ ★

A External carotid

B Greater palatine

C Maxillary

D Posterior ethmoid

E Sphenopalatine

Extended Matching Questions

Causes of head and neck lumps

For each of the following patients with a neck lump, choose the *single* most likely diagnosis from the list below. Each answer can be used once, more than once, or not at all. ★

A Anaplastic carcinoma

B Branchial cyst

C Carotid body tumour

D Dermoid cyst

E Graves' disease

F Hashimoto's thyroiditis

G Lipoma

H Lymphoma

I Multinodular goitre

J Papillary thyroid cancer

K Sebaceous cyst

L Thyroglossal cyst

M Toxoplasmosis

1. A 40-year-old man has multiple soft lymph nodes in the posterior triangle. He has lost weight and has had night sweats for the last 6 weeks.

2. A 15-year-old girl has a painless, midline lump that transilluminates and moves with protrusion of the tongue.

3. An 18-year-old man has a painless lump anterior to the upper third of the sternomastoid on the left. It is under the skin and is soft, fluctuant, and non-tender.

4. A 74-year-old woman has a hard irregular midline lump, difficulty swallowing, and stridor.

5. A 40-year-old woman has a smooth midline lump that moves with swallowing. She has protuberant eyes and a tremor of her hands.

Securing the airway

For each emergency airway scenario, choose the *single* most appropriate initial step to secure the airway from the list of options below. Each option may be used once, more than once, or not at all. ★

A Cricothyroidotomy

B Endotracheal intubation

C Laryngeal mask airway

D Nasal cannulae

E Nasopharyngeal airway

F Nebulized acetylcysteine

G Nebulized adrenaline (epinephrine)

H Nebulized ipratropium

I Nebulized salbutamol

J Oral chlorphenamine

K Oral prednisolone

L Oropharyngeal airway

M Tracheostomy

6. A 66-year-old woman is extubated following an elective thyroid-ectomy. She is still quite sleepy and has no gag reflex. Her airway needs protection while she is taken to the recovery room.

7. A 30-year-old man is having a picnic. He suddenly chokes on his sandwich. His friend attempts the Heimlich manoeuvre but is unsuccessful. When the paramedics arrive the man is deeply cyanosed and loses consciousness.

8. A 3-year-old boy is in respiratory distress with inspiratory stridor, drooling, and tracheal tug.

9. A 25-year-old man is involved in a motor vehicle collision and sustains bilateral maxillary and mandibular fractures. His airway needs protection while his facial fractures heal.

10. A 14-year-old girl is acutely short of breath following a school sports day. She has widespread expiratory wheeze throughout both lung fields.

Causes of nasal obstruction

For each patient, choose the *single* most likely cause of nasal obstruction from the list of options below. Each option may be used once, more than once, or not at all. ★

A Adenoiditis

B Allergic rhinitis

C Aspergilloma

D Atrophic rhinitis

E Candidiasis

F Maxillary sinusitis

G Mucormycosis

H Nasal polyps

I Osteomyelitis

J Rhinitis medicamentosa

K Sarcoidosis

L Tuberculosis

M Vasomotor rhinitis

11. A 56-year-old man who is a wine taster is unable to work due to anosmia. He also has uncontrollable bilateral watery rhinorrhoea and mild asthma.

12. A 3-year-old boy has bilateral mucopurulent rhinorrhoea and halitosis. He is mouth breathing and also has a conductive hearing loss.

13. A 27-year-old man has unilateral purulent rhinorrhoea and left-sided facial pain following a dental extraction.

14. A 23-year-old woman has had a left-sided frontal headache and bilateral purulent rhinorrhoea for 4 weeks. She has a soft mass overlying the left frontal sinus.

15. A 20-year-old man has a cough and severe red indurated nasal crusting that requires debridement. He also has peripheral oedema, with swollen painful fingers.

Causes of facial palsy

For each of the following patients with facial palsy, choose the *single* most likely diagnosis from the list below. Each answer may be used once, more than once, or not at all. ★

A Acute otitis media

B Adenocarcinoma of the parotid

C Cerebral oedema

D Cholesteatoma

E Embolic stroke

F Haemorrhagic stroke

G Herpes simplex virus infection

H Occipital fracture

I Pleomorphic adenoma

J Sarcoidosis

K Secretory otitis media

L Temporal bone fracture

M Varicella zoster virus infection

16. A 10-year-old boy has had pain in the right ear and difficulty hearing for 2 days. He has a temperature of 38.3°C. He now has a right lower motor neuron facial palsy.

17. A 75-year-old man has a hard mass in front of his right tragus and a right lower motor neuron facial palsy.

18. A 35-year-old man has had a road traffic accident. He has a bruise over the mastoid area and a right-sided lower motor neuron facial nerve palsy.

19. A 78-year-old woman has vertigo and difficulty hearing with a right lower motor neuron facial palsy. There are small vesicles in her ear.

20. A 37-year-old man has had painless offensive discharge from his left ear for 10 years. He has difficulty hearing and a lower motor neuron palsy on the left.

Causes of stridor

For each of the following patients with stridor, choose the *single* most likely diagnosis from the list below. Each answer may be used once, more than once, or not at all. ★

A Bilateral vocal cord palsy

B Bronchogenic carcinoma

C Diphtheria

D Infectious mononucleosis

E Laryngeal cleft

F Laryngeal haemangioma

G Laryngeal papilloma

H Laryngomalacia

I Laryngotracheobronchitis (croup)

J Leukoplakia

K Subglottic stenosis

L Supraglottitis

M Vocal cord nodules

21. A 2-week-old boy has stridor that is worse when he is lying on his back. He is pink in air, and is thriving and breastfeeding well.

22. A 75-year-old man has a sudden onset of hoarseness. He has smoked 30 cigarettes a day for 40 years. On examination of the larynx, he has a left-sided vocal cord palsy.

23. A 6-year-old boy has had progressive stridor and voice change for the last 2 months. He is otherwise well and has no temperature.

24. A 70-year-old man is unwell, has difficulty swallowing, and is drooling saliva. He has a temperature of 39°C and a heart rate of 110 bpm.

25. A 2-year-old boy has had a cold for 2 days. He now has a barking cough and a hoarse voice, and has had stridor for 24 hours. He has had two previous similar episodes.

Causes of thyroid pathology

For each clinical scenario, choose the *single* most likely thyroid pathology from the list of options below. Each option may be used once, more than once, or not at all. ★

A Adenoma

B Anaplastic carcinoma

C Follicular carcinoma

D Graves' disease

E Hashimoto's thyroiditis

F Lymphoma

G Medullary carcinoma

H Multinodular goitre

I Papillary carcinoma

J Pyramidal lobe cyst

K Parathyroid adenoma

L Thyroid cyst

M Toxic adenoma

26. A 66-year-old woman has weight loss and palpitations. She has a 2 cm lump in the left lobe of the thyroid, and the rest of the gland is impalpable. There is no palpable cervical lymphadenopathy. Her pulse rate is 100 bpm and it is irregularly irregular.

27. An 84-year-old woman has a rapidly growing irregular hard mass in the anterior triangle of her neck. She also has dysphagia and inspiratory stridor.

28. A 24-year-old woman has a 2 cm lump in the left anterior triangle at the level of the left lobe of the thyroid gland. The skin overlying the lump is normal, and the lump itself is brilliantly transilluminable.

29. A 35-year-old man comes to the Emergency Department with a wrist fracture, after performing a handstand. He has a palpable mass in the left anterior triangle.

30. A 60-year-old woman has fatigue, constipation, and depression. She has diffuse enlargement of the thyroid gland.

ANSWERS

Single Best Answers

1. B ★

About one-third of recurrent laryngeal nerve palsies are caused by cancers, and 40% of these are in the larynx. The risk is increased in smokers. The left recurrent laryngeal nerve has a long course and loops down under the arch of the aorta in the chest, so it may be affected in malignant tumours of the mediastinum. This is less common on the right side. Oesophageal cancers can have pressure effects, but dysphagia would be more prominent.

2. C ★   OHCS 9th edn → p. 540

There is a long history of suppuration here. Chronic suppurative otitis media causes a conductive hearing loss, demonstrated by the tuning fork tests. Otitis externa does not cause mucoid discharge, as the external ear canal does not produce mucus.

3. E ★   OHCS 9th edn → p. 570

A schwannoma, or acoustic neuroma, is a slow-growing benign tumour that causes problems by exerting local pressure on the eighth cranial nerve, which can result in tinnitus and hearing loss. The main differential diagnosis is a meningioma. However, in this location, vestibular schwannomas are more common, although MRI imaging is needed to distinguish them.

4. E ★   OHCS 9th edn → p. 652

This is Ramsay Hunt syndrome, caused by reactivation of varicella zoster virus in a patient who has had chickenpox in the past. The combination of otalgia, hearing impaiment, vertigo, a lower motor neuron facial nerve palsy, and visible vesicles gives the diagnosis.

5. B ★

Crohn's disease causes non-caseating granulomata in the gastrointestinal (GI) tract, anywhere from the mouth to the anus, so should always be a differential diagnosis in any patient with unusual or persistent mouth ulceration, especially when coupled with other GI signs or symptoms. Tuberculosis causes caseating granulomata. Ulcerative colitis affects only the colon, not the upper GI tract.

6. A ★   OHCS 9th edn → pp. 554–555

Benign positional vertigo is common after a head injury. Attacks are provoked by head movement. Labyrinthitis usually follows a viral illness. In Ménière's disease there is associated tinnitus. Temporal bone fracture causes severe dizziness, often associated with facial nerve palsy and hearing loss.

7. D ★

Perforations may heal on their own, but while the drum is perforated there is an increased risk of ear infection, so it is best to keep water out. Sudden loud noises may cause perforations, and surgical closure by means of a myringoplasty operation may be needed later.

8. C ★   OHCS 9th edn → p. 544

This man has a cholesteatoma—that is, an area of skin in the middle ear that is locally destructive. It can be secondary to a tear in the tympanic membrane, and skin grows through. If a patient has chronic discharge, this should be considered. On examination, a cottage-cheese-like discharge is seen. If left untreated, it can invade intracranially, so surgical treatment is needed to remove the sac. A mastoidectomy may be required.

9. E ★   OHCS 9th edn → p. 570

Around 85% of pharyngeal cancers are squamous. Risk factors are smoking or chewing tobacco, and older age, and human papillomavirus infection is also an increasingly common cause.

10. D ★   OHCS 9th edn → p. 568

Hypothyroidism can cause oedema of the vocal cords and therefore hoarseness. The history of lethargy and weight gain adds further clues. Thyroid dysfunction can also cause hoarseness due to pressure from a goitre. The list of causes of hoarseness is long, and therefore you need to look for other clues in the history and examination.

11. A ★

Airway obstruction due to tonsillar hypertrophy is an indication for tonsillectomy. This child's saturations are dipping to 80% during sleep, which indicates significant obstruction. Adenoid and tonsil tissue can be large in young children, and in this situation both need to be removed. Although a Cochrane review has highlighted the fact that there are no good-quality trial data on efficacy, this is still the gold standard treatment when obstruction is demonstrated. If this fails and there are other problems, such as significant obesity or neuromuscular problems, oxygen and CPAP may become necessary, but they are not first-line approaches to management. Similarly, palatal stiffening procedures, such as the insertion of implants, may be used in adults but are not appropriate in growing children.

→ http://summaries.cochrane.org/CD003136/adenotonsillectomy-for-obstructive-sleep-apnoea-in-children

12. E ★

Spores indicate a fungal infection, so an antifungal medication is needed. People who are immunocompromised are at increased risk of such infections. However, oral and IV treatments are not usually necessary as a first-line treatment, and topical treatment should be given in healthy patients. Aluminium acetate can be used as an astringent for otitis externa, but antifungal agents would be better in this proven fungal case.

13. B ★   OHCS 9th edn → p. 544

The high fever, thick purulent discharge, and distorted ear suggest mastoiditis. The ear is typically displaced laterally and inferiorly, and there may be swelling seen over the mastoid process behind the ear. This is a serious infection, and the child should be admitted and given IV antibiotics while surgical treatment is considered. Depending on the degree of damage, different surgical procedures are used to drain the pus.

14. E ★

Bloody discharge indicates a squamous cell carcinoma. The tumour tissue is friable and can bleed easily on contact.

15. D ★★   OHCS 9th edn → p. 558

In any patient with chronic recurrent sinus problems, unusual infections or causes need to be considered. An overgrowth of fungi, usually *Aspergillus* species, can form a ball in the sinuses, usually the maxillary sinus. This will look like a mass filling the sinus on scanning. Polyps look like swellings coming from the lining of the sinus on a CT scan. Allergic polyps commonly occur in the ethmoid sinuses. Angiofibromas are rare, and usually cause some distortion of the sinus on a CT scan; they often cause bleeding. Foreign bodies in the sinuses are rare; they sometimes occur as a result of facial trauma.

16. C ★★   OHCS 9th edn → p. 546

Ventilation tubes, or grommets, are the treatment for glue ear, which is more common in Down's syndrome. Glue ear refers to otitis media with effusion, and is the main cause of hearing loss in young children. This boy has evidence of hearing impairment on his audiograms. If left untreated, this may seriously affect his learning and development.

17. C ★★   OHCS 9th edn → pp. 570–571

Post-cricoid tumours in the hypopharynx often cause the sensation of a lump in the throat before they interfere with swallowing. As they grow, they cause local pain. They can also cause referred pain to the ear along the sensory fibres of the vagus nerve. This is an ominous sign. Clinical anaemia also indicates that the tumour is advanced.

18. C ★★ OHCS 9th edn → p. 552

A glomus tumour, or non-chromaffin paraganglioma, is a rare vascular benign tumour that arises from the glomus body (a small collection of paraganglionic tissue). These tumours often occur in the middle ear. Because of blood flow, the tinnitus is pulsatile. A mass may also be felt in the ear. Glomus tumours can also occur in the carotid body, but would not give these symptoms.

19. B ★★ OHCS 9th edn → p. 568

The cricoarytenoid joints rotate with the vocal cords, so arthritis here causing stiffness can affect the pitch and tone of the voice. This has been reported in 17–70% of patients with rheumatoid arthritis, and airway obstruction by swelling is a rare but serious complication.

20. B ★★ OHCS 9th edn → p. 554

This is a description of Ménière's disease, which involves attacks of disabling vertigo with unilateral tinnitus and progressive sensorineural hearing loss. Treatment is symptomatic initially. Anti-emetics such as cyclizine or prochlorperazine may help to relieve the symptoms but will not reduce the frequency of attacks. Betahistine may be helpful and can be tried, although trial results are equivocal.

21. E ★★ OHCS 9th edn → pp. 540, 546

Fluid in the middle ear causes dampening of the tympanic membrane movement and results in hearing impairment and a flat trace on tympanometry. Serous effusion can occur during the resolution of an acute otitis media, probably due to Eustachian tube dysfunction. It will usually resolve within 3 months. Recurrent infections can lead to a cycle of inflammation, and can cause chronic suppurative otitis media.

22. A ★★ OHCS 9th edn → p. 576

The characteristic appearance of this infection is an enlarging non-tender violaceous mass. It does not disappear following antibiotic use. It is rare, but should be considered.

23. D ★★ OHCS 9th edn → p. 554

The unusual feature here is the intention tremor, which should raise suspicion of a brain lesion. Vertigo caused by central lesions is rare, but features in the history may lead you to suspect these. The other tests assess hearing or assess each labyrinth in turn.

24. B ★ ★

Voice therapy may be all that is required. Surgical approaches employing sharp dissection or laser should only be used if the nodule is resistant to voice therapy. Hypothyroidism is a cause of hoarseness, but not of nodules. Propranolol is used to treat haemangiomata of the larynx, but not nodules.

Surgical versus non-surgical interventions for vocal cord nodules:

→ http://onlinelibrary.wiley.com/doi/10.1002/14651858.CD001934/full

25. **B** ★ ★ ★

The orbital abscess would be seen on CT scan, and any bony defect would be seen on the CT scan but not the MRI scan. A sinus X-ray is very rarely, if ever, performed, and would not show detail of abscess formation. An ultrasound probe could not be used for an abscess in this location, as it is medial to the orbit, and the probe could not be accommodated in the available anatomical space.

Rahbar R et al (2001). Management of orbital subperiosteal abscess in children. *Arch Otolaryngol Head Neck Surg* **127**: 281–286.

26. **B** ★ ★ ★

Children often choke on small foreign bodies, which may become lodged in the airway. If left, they can cause erosion, obstruction, or infection and collapse. Larger objects tend to get stuck in the larynx, and may cause airway obstruction or hoarseness. The majority of foreign bodies get stuck in the bronchus and cause unilateral wheeze and breath sounds, and may cause cough. Without the classic history, these may be missed or mistaken for asthma. Although inspiratory and expiratory chest X-rays may be helpful, very young children cannot cooperate with these, and a single chest film may miss the diagnosis. To look for the foreign body, you need to examine the upper and lower airway carefully by bronchoscopy.

27. **C** ★ ★ ★   OHCS 9th edn → p. 560

Clear fluid that is positive for glucose on a dipstick test suggests a basal skull fracture and leakage of cerebrospinal fluid (CSF). β-2 transferrin is a protein found only in CSF and perilymph, so it can be used to confirm CSF rhinorrhea in suspected basal skull fracture.

28. **A** ★ ★ ★   OHCS 9th edn → p. 560

This boy has a septal haematoma, which is causing the obstruction. The condition is rare but serious, and if left untreated can cause septal necrosis and collapse. Treatment involves draining it under general anaesthesia and packing the nose. Septoplasty or rhinoplasty may be needed later after fractures if the nose sets abnormally and causes deviation of the septum and blockage or deformity.

29. D ★★★ OHCS 9th edn → p. 560

Batteries are corrosive and require urgent removal.

30. C ★★★★

→ www.cancerhelp.org.uk/help/default.asp?page=5647

31. E ★★★★ OHCS 9th edn → p. 563

Ongoing epistaxis despite nasal packing is an emergency, and the nose needs to be examined under anaesthesia. The sphenopalatine artery is a branch of the external carotid artery, and it passes through the sphenopalatine foramen into the back of the nose. It is distal, so ligation usually controls bleeding with few complications. Older techniques involving ligation of the external carotid or maxillary artery have higher complication rates.

Extended Matching Questions

1. H ★

Weight loss, night sweats, and fever are worrying symptoms that you should specifically ask about in any patient with a neck swelling. They are known as the B symptoms in lymphoma.

2. L ★

This is the classic description of a thyroglossal cyst, which is a cystic swelling that develops along the thyroglossal duct.

3. B ★

This is a congenital remnant of embryonic development, resulting from failure of obliteration of the second branchial cleft. These cysts may go unnoticed for some time. The position is typical, between the sternomastoid and the pharynx, and the cyst appears to be fluid-filled.

4. A ★

This is an aggressive form of malignancy that gives a hard tethered goitre, often with surrounding lymphadenopathy, and presses on the surrounding structures.

5. E ★

Graves' disease is an autoimmune thyroiditis. Autoantibodies stimulate thyroid-stimulating hormone receptors and cause increased thyroid hormone production. They also cause a diffuse goitre and inflammation of the tissues in the eyes, leading to exophthalmos. The resulting thyrotoxicosis causes symptoms and signs, including tremor.

General feedback on 1–5: OHCS 9th edn → p. 570

6. L ★

The oropharyngeal (Guedel) airway is suitable for patients with no gag reflex. It is easy to insert and remove.

7. A ★

In confirmed airway obstruction at or above the level of the larynx, cricothyroidotomy is the final step for providing a temporary emergency airway. It can be performed relatively quickly by emergency staff.

8. G ★

In laryngotracheobronchitis in children, nebulized steroid or adrenaline can be used to decrease laryngeal swelling. Oral dexamethasone can also be used, but prednisolone is not appropriate.

9. M ★

In patients with significant facial injuries, airway obstruction can occur because of the swelling, so medium-term ventilation may be needed. A tracheostomy may be more suitable than endotracheal intubation in this case.

10. I ★

The treatment for wheeze is salbutamol, which is a bronchodilatator.

General feedback on 6–10: OHCS 9th edn → pp. 566–567

11. H ★

These cause a watery nasal discharge and post-nasal drip. Changes in the sense of smell are frequent.

12. A ★

Enlarged adenoids are common in children, and can lead to mouth breathing, snoring, and bad breath due to airway obstruction. Inflammatory mediators from the adenoidal tissue cause swelling and blockage of the Eustachian tubes, which can lead to dysfunction and fluid in the middle ear.

13. F ★

Dental root infection can spread to the sinuses and cause a foul-smelling discharge and cheek pain.

14. I ★

This is uncommon, but the prolonged history of purulent discharge suggests bacterial infection. Such a mass would be uncommon in simple sinusitis. This is also called a Pott's puffy tumour.

15. K ★

Sarcoid skin plaques often appear on the face. The collection of unusual signs and symptoms in this patient should point towards a systemic disorder. Tuberculosis can cause cough, but would not cause the same plaque-like rash and finger swelling.

General feedback on 11–15: OHCS 9th edn → pp. 556, 561

16. A ★

Infection in the middle ear can spread to the facial nerve. Acute otitis media is common in children, although this complication is unusual. In 6% of the population the bony canal that carries the facial nerve in the middle ear is dehiscent, and consequently middle ear infection can cause facial palsy in these individuals.

17. B ★

The parotid gland lies in front of the tragus and curves around the angle of the mandible. Malignant tumours are rare (80% of masses are pleomorphic adenomas), but the hard texture and invasion to cause a nerve VII palsy suggest this.

18. L ★

The trauma here suggests a fracture. Around 50% of transverse temporal bone fractures will result in some facial paralysis.

19. M ★

Varicella zoster virus can infect cranial nerves VII and VIII, causing facial paralysis, ear pain, vertigo, and hearing loss.

20. D ★

This is a serious condition, caused by skin in the middle ear and mastoid that is locally destructive. The discharge may be ignored, and patients often present late with headache, pain, facial paralysis, and vertigo as the cholesteatoma erodes. Treatment is by surgery.

General feedback on 16–20: OHCS 9th edn → pp. 542–544, 570, 578

21. H ★

This is the commonest cause of stridor in neonates. Babies are usually well and feed without problems, but the stridor can be very loud and may cause alarm. It is due to shortened aryepiglottic folds and immature floppy cartilage, which cause the larynx to collapse on inspiration.

22. B ★

Lung cancer can cause a recurrent laryngeal nerve palsy. The nerve descends into the chest before passing back up to innervate the intrinsic muscles of the larynx.

23. G ★

The chronic progressive nature suggests that this is not an acute infection, which would be the commonest cause in children. Laryngeal papillomas are similar to warts on the larynx, caused by human papillomavirus, and they usually occur in children.

24. L ★

This acute history in a toxic patient suggests infection. Supraglottitis is uncommon but is life-threatening. The inability to swallow even saliva suggests airway obstruction.

25. I ★

Croup, or viral laryngotracheobronchitis, is a common illness in children under the age of about 7 years. It is usually preceded by a cold, and progresses to a typical barking cough and stridor. It can be recurrent.

General feedback on 21–25: OHCS 9th edn → pp. 566–568

26. M ★

A thyroid adenoma is a benign solitary tumour. It can be silent, but may produce thyroxine and cause symptoms of hyperthyroidism. In contrast, a multinodular goitre results in a diffusely lumpy gland.

27. B ★

This is an aggressive form of malignancy that gives a hard tethered goitre, often with surrounding lymphadenopathy, and presses on the surrounding structures.

28. L ★

A cyst is a fluid-filled lump, so it will transilluminate.

29. K ★

A parathyroid adenoma will produce parathyroid hormone, which causes calcium resorption from bone by indirectly stimulating osteoclasts. It can therefore present with fractures caused by minimal trauma.

30. E ★

These are symptoms of hypothyroidism. Hashimoto's thyroiditis is an autoimmune disease and is the commonest cause of hypothyroidism. The gland swells as a result of being diffusely invaded by inflammatory cells.

Chapter 7

Dermatology

Virginia Hubbard

Skin disease has a serious impact on an individual's quality of life. It is well recognized that conditions such as psoriasis may have a similar impact on a patient's quality of life to chronic diseases such as diabetes, hypertension, and depression.

Skin problems account for approximately 20% of all patient consultations in primary care in the UK. It is important that clinicians are able to diagnose common skin diseases such as acne, eczema, psoriasis, and cutaneous malignancies, and initiate an appropriate management plan. This requires the ability to take a full history and conduct a complete examination. A complete dermatological examination involves examination of the entire skin, mucous membranes, hair, and nails. The description of cutaneous pathologies should include the location and distribution of lesions. The morphology of a lesion or each component of a generalized eruption should be noted. Other organ systems may also need to be examined.

The questions in this chapter will test your knowledge of the skin problems that are frequently encountered in non-specialist clinical practice. Other more rare skin disorders are also covered, either because they are potentially life-threatening or because they are a sign of systemic disease. The questions are designed to improve your ability to recognize the morphology and distribution of cutaneous physical signs.

Hopefully you will find these questions stimulating and an aid to improving your knowledge of skin disease.

QUESTIONS

Single Best Answers

1. A 42-year-old man with type 2 diabetes has hyperpigmented skin in his axillae, as shown in Plate 7.1 (see Colour Plate section). Which is the single most likely diagnosis? ★

A Acanthosis nigricans

B Atopic eczema

C Erythrasma

D Seborrhoeic dermatitis

E Tinea corporis

2. A 28-year-old man has had red scaly patches over his cheeks, as shown in Plate 7.2 (see Colour Plate section), for 2 years. He also has scaling of the skin around his eyebrows. Which is the single most likely diagnosis? ★

A Atopic eczema

B Candidiasis

C Psoriasis

D Seborrhoeic dermatitis

E Tinea faciei

3. A 14-year-old girl has lesions on her fingers, as shown in Plate 7.3 (see Colour Plate section). They have been present for 5 months. Which is the single most likely causative organism? ★

A Adenovirus

B Coxsackievirus

C Herpes simplex virus

D Human papillomavirus

E Molluscum contagiosum virus

4. A 23-year-old woman has a rash affecting her forehead, cheeks, and chin, as shown in Plate 7.4 (see Colour Plate section). Which is the single predominant lesion shown here? ★

A Comedone

B Macule

C Nodule

D Papule

E Pustule

5. A 30-year-old woman has had itchy skin for most of her life. Her face is shown in Plate 7.5 (see Colour Plate section). Which is the single most likely diagnosis? ★

A Acne rosacea

B Atopic eczema

C Impetigo

D Psoriasis

E Seborrhoeic dermatitis

6. A 38-year-old woman with lifelong atopic eczema has noticed that her eczema has been getting worse over the past 7 days. She has been taking flucloxacillin for 4 days, but her condition is worsening, as shown in Plate 7.6 (see Colour Plate section), and is becoming painful. Which single treatment should be given? ★

A Betamethasone valerate ointment

B Emulsifying ointment

C IV aciclovir

D IV benzylpenicillin

E Oral metronidazole

7. A 36-year-old man has had a skin rash, as shown in Plate 7.7 (see Colour Plate section), for 20 years. Which is the single most likely diagnosis? ★

A Atopic eczema

B Lichen planus

C Pityriasis versicolor

D Psoriasis

E Seborrhoeic dermatitis

8. A 40-year-old woman attends her GP surgery for a Well Woman check-up. She has multiple skin lesions, as shown in Plate 7.8 (see Colour Plate section), that have been present since she was a child and are slowly increasing in number. Which is the single most likely diagnosis? ★

A Epidermoid cysts

B Ganglions

C Neurofibromatosis

D Tuberous sclerosis

E Viral warts

9. A 56-year-old man presents with a thumb that appears as shown in Plate 7.9 (see Colour Plate section). He jammed the thumb in a door a few months ago. The rest of his skin examination is normal. Which is the single most likely diagnosis? ★

A Haematoma

B Lichen planus

C Malignant melanoma

D Onychomycosis

E Psoriasis

10. A 37-year-old woman has painful swollen distal interpharyngeal joints. She has the nail changes shown in Plate 7.10 (see Colour Plate section), and says that her nails have been like this for 10 years. Which is the single most likely diagnosis? ★

A Atopic eczema

B Lichen planus

C Psoriasis

D Systemic lupus erythematosus

E Tinea manuum

11. A 40-year-old woman has had a swollen leg for 6 days, as shown in Plate 7.11 (see Colour Plate section). Her temperature is 38.6°C and her full blood count shows a neutrophil count of 11×10^9/L. Which is the single most likely diagnosis? ★

A Cellulitis

B Deep vein thrombosis

C Psoriasis

D Tinea corporis

E Venous eczema

12. A 40-year-old man has skin between his toes, as shown in Plate 7.12 (see Colour Plate section). Which is the single most likely diagnosis? ★

A Atopic eczema

B Candidiasis

C Psoriasis

D Tinea pedis

E Viral wart

13. A 5-year-old girl has had blisters on her left thigh, as shown in Plate 7.13 (see Colour Plate section), for 2 days. The condition started with a yellow crusted area 5 days ago, which spread, and then the blisters appeared. The girl is otherwise well. Which is the single most likely diagnosis? ★

A Bullous impetigo

B Bullous pemphigoid

C Chronic bullous disease of childhood

D Insect bites

E Scabies

14. A 35-year-old woman has had a skin problem for a number of years. She had a Caesarean section last year, and her scar is shown in Plate 7.14 (see Colour Plate section). Which is the single best description of the appearance? ★

A Auspitz sign

B Impetiginization

C Keloid scar

D Köbner phenomenon

E Striae

15. A 34-year-old man has a lesion on his leg, as shown in Plate 7.15 (see Colour Plate section). He first noticed it about 2 months ago. Which is the single most likely diagnosis? ★

A Actinic keratosis

B Benign naevus

C Bowen's disease

D Malignant melanoma

E Seborrhoeic keratosis

16. A 10-month-old baby has had skin lesions, as shown in Plate 7.16 (see Colour Plate section), for 2 days. He had an upper respiratory tract infection last week, but seems to be well in himself now. The lesions appear to be in a different place from the ones he had yesterday. Which is the single most likely diagnosis? ★

A Acute urticaria

B Atopic eczema

C Erythema multiforme

D Meningococcal septicaemia

E Urticaria pigmentosa

17. A 28-year-old woman developed a rash on her body 1 week ago. Today it has spread to her hands, as shown in Plate 7.17 (see Colour Plate section). Three weeks ago she had a 3-day course of trimethoprim to treat a urinary tract infection. Which is the single most likely diagnosis? ★

A Acute urticaria

B Allergic contact eczema

C Erythema multiforme

D Erythema nodosum

E Psoriasis

18. A 64-year-old man has had a sore back and mouth for 2 months. These are shown in Plate 7.18 (a, b) (see Colour Plate section). Which is the single most likely diagnosis? ★

A Bullous pemphigoid

B Erythema multiforme

C Herpes simplex virus infection

D Lichen planus

E Pemphigus vulgaris

19. A 30-year-old man with ulcerative colitis has lesions on his anterior shins. The lesions started to develop 7 months ago and are getting bigger. They are shown in Plate 7.19 (see Colour Plate section). Which is the single most likely diagnosis? ★

A Erythema nodosum

B Leucocytoclastic vasculitis

C Necrobiosis lipoidica

D Pyoderma gangrenosum

E Venous ulcers

20. A 60-year-old man has a lesion on his arm that has grown rapidly over the past 3 weeks, and that is not painful. It is shown in Plate 7.20 (see Colour Plate section). Which is the single most likely diagnosis? ★

A Actinic keratosis

B Basal-cell carcinoma

C Keratoacanthoma

D Malignant melanoma

E Seborrhoeic keratosis

21. A 22-year-old man has a lesion on his lower abdomen that is increasing in size, and which is shown in Plate 7.21 (see Colour Plate section). He has tried 1% hydrocortisone cream to no avail. Which is the single most appropriate treatment? ★

A Betamethasone valerate cream

B Ketoconazole shampoo

C Oral flucloxacillin

D Oral prednisolone

E Oral terbinafine

22. A 45-year-old man had a cardiac transplant 8 years ago. He has developed a painful lesion on his forehead that is irregular in shape with a thick crust. The lesion has grown rapidly over the past 3 months. Which is the single most likely diagnosis? ★

A Actinic keratosis

B Bowen's disease

C Malignant melanoma

D Seborrhoeic keratosis

E Squamous cell carcinoma

23. An 18-year-old man has severe scarring acne with multiple nodules and cysts on his face, which has been getting progressively worse over the past 5 years. Treatment with oxytetracycline for 8 months has not helped. He is otherwise well. Which is the single most appropriate treatment? ★

A 5% Benzoyl peroxide cream

B Clobetasone butyrate cream

C Oral erythromycin

D Oral isotretinoin

E Oral prednisolone

24. A 3-month-old baby has a rash on his groin. He is otherwise well. The rash is shown in Plate 7.22 (see Colour Plate section). Which is the single most appropriate treatment to prescribe? ★

A 1% Hydrocortisone cream

B Aqueous cream

C Fucidin cream

D No treatment

E Nystatin cream

25. A 56-year-old woman has a sore red dry itchy rash that is confined to her face. It has developed over the past month. The rest of her skin is normal. She is otherwise well and is taking no medication. Which is the single most likely diagnosis? ★

A Acne rosacea

B Allergic contact dermatitis

C Atopic eczema

D Seborrhoeic dermatitis

E Systemic lupus erythematosus

26. The nose of a 69-year-old man has the appearance shown in Plate 7.23 (see Colour Plate section). It has looked like this for 9 years. Which is the single best term to describe the appearance? ★ ★

A Acne vulgaris

B Lupus pernio

C Lupus vulgaris

D Rhinophyma

E Wegener's granulomatosis

27. A 26-year-old man with atopic eczema has lesions on his palms, as shown in Plate 7.24 (see Colour Plate section), which are very itchy. They come and go, and seem to flare up when the rest of his eczema is bad. He has not yet tried any treatments as he is unsure which of them to use. Which is the single most appropriate treatment? ★ ★

A 1% Hydrocortisone ointment

B 5% Permethrin cream

C Aciclovir cream

D Betamethasone valerate ointment

E Ketoconazole cream

28. A 12-year-old boy has had atopic eczema for many years. He is concerned about paler patches on his face, shown in Plate 7.25 (see Colour Plate section), which have been present for the past 6 months. He has changes consistent with eczema over the rest of his skin, but no pigmentary change. Which is the single most likely diagnosis? ★ ★

A Cutaneous T-cell lymphoma

B Pityriasis alba

C Seborrhoeic dermatitis

D Tinea faciei

E Vitiligo

29. A 78-year-old woman has an itchy rash over her trunk and limbs, as shown in Plate 7.26 (see Colour Plate section). She has been itchy for several weeks, and blisters appeared last week. She is not taking any regular medication. Which is the single most likely diagnosis? ★ ★

A Bullous pemphigoid

B Erythema multiforme

C Pemphigus vulgaris

D Psoriasis

E Scabies

30. A 47-year-old man has had a rash over both lower legs for 2 days, as shown in Plate 7.27 (see Colour Plate section). He was treated with amoxicillin for a throat infection last week. Which is the single most likely diagnosis? ★ ★

A Cellulitis

B Erythema multiforme

C Erythema nodosum

D Leukocytoclastic vasculitis

E Streptococcal septicaemia

31. A 36-year-old woman is concerned about the pigmentation on her cheeks, shown in Plate 7.28 (see Colour Plate section), which is spreading. She is not taking any medication. Which is the single most appropriate treatment? ★ ★

A Betamethasone valerate cream

B High-factor sunblock

C Hydroquinone cream

D Hydroxychloroquine

E Oral prednisolone for 6 weeks

32. A 30-year-old woman gave birth 7 weeks ago. She has had a lesion on her breast for 2 weeks. It bleeds profusely and interferes with breastfeeding of her baby. Which is the single most likely diagnosis? ★ ★

A Bacillary angiomatosis

B Granuloma annulare

C Pyoderma gangrenosum

D Pyogenic granuloma

E Viral wart

33. A 30-year-old man has been on a walking holiday in Spain and now has blisters, shown in Plate 7.29 (see Colour Plate section). The remainder of his skin is normal. Which is the single most likely diagnosis? ★ ★

A Allergic contact eczema

B Bullous pemphigoid

C Impetigo

D Insect bite reaction

E Linear IgA disease

34. An 18-month-old girl has a widespread rash on her trunk. It started to develop 2 weeks ago with a single round red plaque 2 cm in diameter on her left flank. This was treated with topical anti-fungal cream, with no effect. During the last 3 days several more scaly plaques have appeared over the trunk. These are 1 cm in diameter, and pink in the centre with a dark red ring around the outside. They are itchy. The girl is well in herself and is thriving. Which is the single most likely diagnosis? ★ ★ ★

A Guttate psoriasis

B Pityriasis rosea

C Seborrhoeic dermatitis

D Tinea corporis

E Viral exanthema

Extended Matching Questions

Extended Matching Questions

Causes of skin lumps

For each patient with a skin lesion, choose the *single* most likely diagnosis from the list of options below. Each option may be used once, more than once, or not at all. ★

A Basal-cell carcinoma

B Becker's naevus

C Benign intradermal naevus

D Dermatofibroma

E Malignant melanoma

F Pilomatricoma

G Seborrhoeic keratosis

H Squamous cell carcinoma

1. A 74-year-old woman has a lesion on her nose. It has been present for 6 months. It bleeds and crusts but never clears, and is shown in Plate 7.30 (see Colour Plate section).

2. A 47-year-old woman noticed a lesion on her abdomen 3 months ago. It is itchy, has not changed in appearance, and is shown in Plate 7.31 (see Colour Plate section).

3. A 30-year-old woman noticed a lesion on her calf shortly after returning from holiday in Cyprus. It is shown in Plate 7.32 (see Colour Plate section).

4. A 35-year-old man has a lesion on his back. It was first noticed by his wife, who has been asking him to show it to a doctor because it has been increasing in size over the past 2 months. The lesion is shown in Plate 7.33 (see Colour Plate section).

5. A 14-year-old boy has a lesion on his shoulder. It appeared at puberty, and it causes him embarrassment when he is changing for sport. It is shown in Plate 7.34 (see Colour Plate section).

Causes of skin infections

For each patient with a rash, choose the *single* most likely causative organism from the list of options below. Each option may be used once, more than once, or not at all. ★

A *Borrelia burgdorferi*

B *Clostridium botulinum*

C *Escherichia coli*

D Herpes simplex virus

E Molluscum contagiosum virus

F *Sarcoptes scabiei*

G *Staphylococcus aureus*

H Varicella zoster virus

6. A 32-year-old woman with type 1 diabetes has a hot red painful leg, which is shown in Plate 7.35 (see Colour Plate section).

7. An 8-year-old girl has developed lesions around her mouth over the past 4 days, which are shown in Plate 7.36 (see Colour Plate section).

8. A 5-year-old boy has lesions on his abdomen that have been present for about 1 month. His father reports that new lesions are developing. They are shown in Plate 7.37 (see Colour Plate section).

9. A 30-year-old woman has had very itchy hands for 1 week. She has no previous history of skin disease. The rash is shown in Plate 7.38 (see Colour Plate section).

10. A 45-year-old man has had a painful rash on his right buttock only for 3 days. It is shown in Plate 7.39 (see Colour Plate section).

Causes of itchy or painful rashes

For each patient with an itchy or painful rash, choose the *single* most likely diagnosis from the list of options below. Each option may be used once, more than once, or not at all. ★

A Bullous impetigo

B Bullous pemphigoid

C Dermatitis herpetiformis

D Lichen planus

E Pemphigus vulgaris

F Tinea capitis

G Tinea corporis

H Varicella zoster virus

11. A 28-year-old woman with hepatitis C has a very itchy rash over the volar aspect of her wrists, as shown in Plate 7.40 (see Colour Plate section). The rash also affects her ankles.

12. A 34-year-old man with coeliac disease has very itchy lesions over his buttocks, as shown in Plate 7.41 (see Colour Plate section). He has a similar rash over his elbows and knees.

13. A 75-year-old man has been experiencing itching for 2 months. Over the past 2 weeks he has developed lesions, as shown in Plate 7.42 (see Colour Plate section).

14. A 44-year-old man has painful blisters over his left arm, as shown in Plate 7.43 (see Colour Plate section). The remainder of his skin is unaffected.

15. A 67-year-old woman has eroded areas of skin on her trunk. Her mouth is very sore and has ulcers, as shown in Plate 7.44 (see Colour Plate section).

Causes of scaly rashes

For each patient, choose the *single* most likely diagnosis from the list of options below. Each option may be used once, more than once, or not at all. ★

A Atopic eczema

B Erythema multiforme

C Erythema nodosum

D Lichen planus

E Pityriasis rosea

F Pityriasis versicolor

G Psoriasis

H Tinea corporis

16. A 34-year-old man has a rash, as shown in Plate 7.45 (see Colour Plate section). He has had a similar rash for 20 years, but it has recently become much worse.

17. A 30-year-old woman has lesions over her trunk, palms, and soles, as shown in Plate 7.46 (see Colour Plate section). She had a cold sore on her lip the previous week.

18. A 12-year-old girl has non-itchy lesions on her arm, as shown in Plate 7.47 (see Colour Plate section). The rash started as a solitary lesion, but two more lesions have since developed.

19. A 20-year-old woman has a scaly scalp, as shown in Plate 7.48 (see Colour Plate section). She also has scaly lesions over her elbows.

20. A 36-year-old woman has had an itchy rash for most of her life. It has been particularly severe over the past month, and is shown in Plate 7.49 (see Colour Plate section).

Drug treatments in skin disorders

For each patient with a rash, choose the *single* most appropriate treatment from the list of options below. Each option may be used once, more than once, or not at all. ★ ★

A Clobetasone butyrate

B Clobetasol propionate

C Ketoconazole shampoo

D Oral chlorphenamine

E Oral griseofulvin

F Oral non-steroidal anti-inflammatory drug

G Oral prednisolone

H Oral tetracycline

21. A 30-year-old woman has had a rash for 2 months. It is shown in Plate 7.50 (see Colour Plate section).

22. A 24-year-old woman is on the oral contraceptive pill, but is not taking any other medications. She has developed painful lumps on her shins, which are shown in Plate 7.51 (see Colour Plate section).

23. A 50-year-old man has had lesions on his face, which are shown in Plate 7.52 (see Colour Plate section), for 14 months. He has tried potent topical corticosteroids, which helped initially, but then the spots became worse. The remainder of his skin is unaffected.

24. An 8-year-old girl has developed a boggy mass on her scalp, shown in Plate 7.53 (see Colour Plate section). For the past 3 months she has had areas of hair loss that have been diagnosed as ringworm.

25. A 24-year-old man has tan-coloured patches on his trunk, which are shown in Plate 7.54 (see Colour Plate section). They appeared in the summer, and are not itchy.

Causes of hair and skin disorders

For each patient, choose the *single* most likely diagnosis from the list of options below. Each option may be used once, more than once, or not at all. ★ ★

A Acne keloidalis nuchae

B Alopecia areata

C Androgenetic alopecia

D Discoid lupus erythematosus

E Pityriasis alba

F Systemic lupus erythematosus

G Tinea capitis

H Vitiligo

26. A 38-year-old woman has noticed that her hair has been thinning over the past year. Her thyroid function and ferritin levels are normal. Her scalp is shown in Plate 7.55 (see Colour Plate section).

27. A 33-year-old man has three discrete bald patches, one of which is shown in Plate 7.56 (see Colour Plate section). These have developed over the past 3 months. There has been no trauma to the scalp and he is otherwise well.

28. A 55-year-old woman has a patch of hair loss over the parietal region, which is shown in Plate 7.57 (see Colour Plate section). This has developed over the past 6 months. She also has atrophic erythematous plaques over her ears.

29. A 5-year-old boy has lost hair in patches over his scalp. This has progressed over the past 6 weeks. His scalp is shown in Plate 7.58 (see Colour Plate section).

30. A 25-year-old man has had gradual loss of all of his hair. This started as two small bald patches, but subsequently spread to involve all of the hair on his head. He has also lost his eyebrows, eyelashes, and axillary hair. He is otherwise well and is not taking any medication. His scalp is shown in Plate 7.59 (see Colour Plate section).

ANSWERS

Single Best Answers

1. A ★   OHCS 9th edn → p. 588

This condition is more common in patients with type 2 diabetes. It causes velvety hyperpigmented plaques in the axillae, groin, and neck folds.

2. D ★   OHCS 9th edn → p. 596

This common dermatosis causes scaling and erythema in the nasolabial folds, eyebrows, and hairline. There may be associated fine scale on the scalp and within the ears.

3. D ★   OHCS 9th edn → p. 599

These are viral warts, caused by human papillomavirus.

4. E ★   OHCS 9th edn → p. 584

5. B ★   OHCS 9th edn → p. 596

Atopic eczema is classically itchy, and it typically affects flexural sites. It is common for there to be facial involvement, as seen here.

6. C ★   OHCS 9th edn → p. 599

This is eczema herpeticum (eczema infected with herpes simplex virus). Note the characteristic monomorphic vesicles. The history of the eczema getting worse despite antibiotic treatment is a clue. This infection spreads very quickly and requires IV treatment.

7. D ★   OHCS 9th edn → p. 594

Note the symmetrical distribution of plaques with a silvery scale on the surface. The extensor aspects of the elbows are involved—a classic site for psoriasis.

8. B ★

This is neurofibromatosis type 1. It is an autosomal dominant condition. The multiple dome-shaped tumours are neurofibromas. There may also be café au lait macules and axillary freckling of the skin.

→ www.nfauk.org (Neurofibromatosis Association)

9. C ★   OHCS 9th edn → p. 592

This is an acral subungual melanoma. Note the pigmentation of the skin around the nail (Hutchinson's sign). The nail has been distorted by the growth of the melanoma under the nail bed.

10. C ★   OHCS 9th edn → p. 594

The severe nail dystrophy, swollen distal interphalangeal joints, and fine scaling over the fingertips are suggestive of psoriasis. Approximately 5% of patients with psoriasis develop arthropathy.

11. A ★

A patient with a hot red swollen leg may have cellulitis or a deep vein thrombosis. In this case, the raised temperature, the sharp demarcation of the erythema at the ankle, and the neutrophilia support the diagnosis of cellulitis.

12. D ★   OHCS 9th edn → p. 598

This is 'athlete's foot.' Note the macerated and scaled appearance of the skin in the web space.

13. A ★   OHCS 9th edn → p. 598

Impetigo can cause tense blisters, as shown here. Note the yellow crusted patches, which are more typical of impetigo seen in children.

14. D ★   OHCS 9th edn → p. 584

The Köbner phenomenon describes the occurrence of skin lesions in areas of trauma or surgery. It occurs with psoriasis (as seen here), warts, vitiligo, and lichen planus.

15. D ★   OHCS 9th edn → p. 592

Note the irregular colour of and edge to this lesion. Remember the ABCDE for pigmented lesions:

Asymmetry
Border
Colour
Diameter > 7 mm
Evolution

16. A ★   OHCS 9th edn → p. 603

These are wheals. The history of them being present for less than 24 hours is typical. Acute urticaria can result from infection, drugs, or a food allergy, but often no cause is found.

17. C ★   OHCS 9th edn → p. 588

The targetoid lesions are typical of erythema multiforme. This usually starts on the trunk and spreads acrally (to the hands, feet, and head). Common causes are drugs and infection (typically herpes simplex virus or mycoplasma infection).

18. E ★   OHCS 9th edn → p. 602

Note the eroded areas from superficial blisters that have burst. This is typical of pemphigus vulgaris. The skin around the eroded areas is normal (in contrast, in bullous pemphigoid it is erythematous). The erosions on the lip further support the diagnosis of pemphigus vulgaris.

19. D ★   OHCS 9th edn → p. 588

This condition is more common in patients with inflammatory bowel disease. Note the ulcers with a purple-red border. The ulcers often appear undermined at the edge. Surgical intervention will make this condition worse and may lead to limb amputation, so do not cut these lesions out!

20. C ★   OHCS 9th edn → p. 590

This nodule is growing rapidly and has a symmetrical shape with a central plug of keratin. These lesions are usually excised in order to differentiate them from a squamous cell carcinoma.

21. E ★   OHCS 9th edn → p. 598

This is tinea corporis. It has been exacerbated by the topical steroid that this patient has used. An oral antifungal agent is needed.

22. E ★   OHCS 9th edn → p. 590

This describes an exophytic tumour with a hyperkeratotic crust on a sun-exposed site. Squamous cell carcinoma is more common in organ-transplant recipients as a result of immunosuppressive medication, so must always be considered.

23. D ★   OHCS 9th edn → p. 600

For severe acne, isotretinoin for 16 weeks is the drug of choice. However, close supervision is required, as it has significant side-effects.

24. **E** ★   OHCS 9th edn → p. 598

The satellite pustules that are visible are characteristic of candidiasis. The folds are involved (which makes an extrinsic dermatitis, such as irritant dermatitis, unlikely). This infection is treated with an antifungal cream such as nystatin.

25. **B** ★   OHCS 9th edn → p. 596

The distribution of this eruption gives the clue that this is allergic contact eczema—the eczema is limited to one body site. The face is a common site to be affected by allergic contact dermatitis (common allergens are make-up and hair dye).

26. **D** ★★   OHCS 9th edn → p. 600

This bulbous swelling of the nose has occurred as a result of long-standing rosacea. The tissues have been infiltrated by granulomatous inflammation.

27. **D** ★★

This is pompholyx hand eczema. It consists of very itchy vesicles and papules on the palms. Scabies is less likely in this patient, because the papules come and go together with the rest of his eczema. This form of eczema requires treatment with a potent topical corticosteroid, such as betamethasone valerate.

28. **B** ★★   OHCS 9th edn → p. 586

The patches here have an indistinct border and are hypopigmented (not sharp-edged and depigmented, as would be seen in vitiligo). This is pityriasis alba, which occurs on the faces of children with atopic eczema. It improves with treatment with emollients and mild topical corticosteroid creams.

29. **A** ★★   OHCS 9th edn → p. 602

Note the tense blisters on an erythematous urticated base. Bullous pemphigoid does not usually affect the mucosal membranes.

30. **D** ★★   OHCS 9th edn → p. 588

This is a small-vessel vasculitis causing palpable purpura of the skin. This was the result of a hypersensitivity reaction to amoxicillin. Whenever purpura is seen, it is important to think of systemic sepsis. However, this man is well and has too long a history for this to be the diagnosis.

31. B ★★

This is melasma. The safest treatment is to advise the daily use of a sunblock. Sunshine makes this condition worse. Some women develop melasma while pregnant or when taking the oral contraceptive pill. Hydroquinone can be damaging to the skin, especially at high strength.

32. D ★★   OHCS 9th edn → p. 602

This is a benign vascular tumour that is more common in pregnancy. Lesions are often triggered by trauma.

33. D ★★

Note the tense blisters in this case. The surrounding skin is normal, which makes bullous pemphigoid, linear IgA disease, and allergic contact eczema unlikely. There is no evidence of impetigo here.

34. B ★★★   OHCS 9th edn → p. 586

This is a fairly typical description of pityriasis rosea. The condition starts with a herald patch, which is the key to diagnosis. This is a round plaque 1–2 cm in diameter with a pink centre separated from a dark red edge by a fine scaly area. One to two weeks later a secondary rash appears which is usually on the trunk in a symmetrical distribution. These lesions look like smaller versions of the herald patch, and the rash is usually itchy. Guttate psoriasis is very unusual in young children, and tends to form drop-like salmon-pink lesions with a fine scale. Seborrhoeic dermatitis causes dry flaky skin, often on the scalp, but it can occur in folds and flexural areas. Tinea is a fungal infection and it usually responds to anti-fungal agents. A single red inflamed patch tends to keep growing, with the outer edge more inflamed like a ring. Viral exanthemata are typically erythematous maculopapular rashes that occur with a viral upper respiratory infection.

Extended Matching Questions

1. A ★

This glassy nodule has a rolled edge, typical of a basal-cell carcinoma. The face is the site most commonly affected by a basal-cell carcinoma.

2. G ★

The warty surface of this plaque is typical of a seborrhoeic keratosis. Note the 'stuck-on' appearance.

3. D ★

This regular pink nodule has the characteristic 'button-hole' sign around the edge. Dermatofibromas commonly arise on the lower legs after an insect bite.

4. E ★

The history of this lesion increasing in size should be regarded as a warning that this is a melanoma. The irregular asymmetrical shape and edge with more than three different colours is highly suggestive of malignant melanoma.

5. B ★

This is a form of birthmark that typically occurs at puberty. The shoulder is the characteristic site involved. A Becker's naevus often becomes more hairy over time.

General feedback on 1–5: OHCS 9th edn → pp. 590–592

6. G ★

This is cellulitis. It is caused by organisms that enter the body through a cut in the skin. It is important to take blood cultures and skin swabs. The other common organism that causes cellulitis is *Streptococcus*.

7. G ★

This is impetigo, which commonly starts around the nose and mouth, with a yellow crust on an erythematous base. It is most commonly caused by *Staphylococcus*, and is relatively common in children.

8. E ★

These are umbilicated papules in a cluster, typical of molluscum contagiosum virus infection. This is caused by a pox virus and is highly contagious.

9. F ★

This is scabies. The presence of itchy papules in the web spaces is characteristic of this condition. Burrows may also be seen.

10. H ★

This dermatomal collection of vesicles is characteristic of varicella zoster virus infection (herpes zoster or shingles).

General feedback on 6–10: OHCS 9th edn → pp. 598–599

11. D ★

This is an inflammatory dermatosis that causes very itchy lichenoid papules (note the increased skin markings). Lichen planus is more common in patients infected with hepatitis C virus.

12. C ★

These extremely itchy vesiculopapular lesions affecting the extensor aspects are suggestive of dermatitis herpetiformis. This rash occurs in patients with gluten-sensitive enteropathy, and the rash improves if the patient switches to a gluten-free diet.

13. B ★

The tense dome-shaped blisters on an erythematous base are typical of bullous pemphigoid. This condition is more common in elderly patients. The itching often precedes the blisters.

14. H ★

The dermatomal distribution of the vesicles is the clue to this diagnosis.

15. E ★

Pemphigus vulgaris causes superficial blisters that burst easily, leaving erosions (in contrast to the deeper tense bullae in bullous pemphigoid). Pemphigus vulgaris commonly involves the mucosal membranes, including the mouth, causing erosions and ulcers.

General feedback on 11–15: OHCS 9th edn → pp. 588, 599, 602

16. G ★

Note the erythematous plaques, with a silvery scale on the surface, which are affecting the extensor aspects of the patient's body.

17. B ★

These are target lesions, seen in erythema multiforme, which is most commonly triggered by drugs or by herpes simplex virus infection.

18. H ★

These are the characteristic annular scaly patches of ringworm (tinea corporis).

19. G ★

Psoriasis typically causes plaques over the extensor aspects of the body. It can also affect the scalp, nails, and joints.

20. A ★

Note the flexural distribution of scaly excoriated patches. This is severe eczema.

General feedback on 16–20: OHCS 9th edn → pp. 588, 594–597

---

21. H ★★

This is acne vulgaris. Note the multiple pustules. The most appropriate treatment is with a tetracycline drug.

22. F ★★

This is erythema nodosum, and it was precipitated by the oral contraceptive pill. The appropriate treatment is rest, non-steroidal anti-inflammatory drugs (NSAIDs), and finding an alternative form of contraception.

23. H ★★

This is acne rosacea, which has been made worse by the use of topical corticosteroids. It is treated with oral tetracyclines for at least 4 months.

24. E ★★

This is a kerion, which occurs as part of the host's response to a fungal infection. It should be treated with an oral antifungal agent, such as griseofulvin or terbinafine, for at least 2 weeks. It should not be incised or drained.

25. C ★★

This is pityriasis versicolor, which is caused by a yeast infection on the skin surface. It is treated by using ketoconazole shampoo as a body wash for 1 to 2 weeks to control the scaliness. The pigmentation may take some time to recover. This condition often recurs.

General feedback on 21–25: OHCS 9th edn → pp. 588, 598, 600

---

26. C ★★

There is diffuse non-scarring thinning of the hair. The scalp skin appears normal. This pattern of thinning over the vertex is consistent with the diagnosis of androgenetic alopecia in a female patient.

27. B ★★

There are focal patches of non-scarring alopecia. At the periphery there are exclamation-mark hairs (hairs that become narrower along the length of the strand closer to the base, producing a characteristic 'exclamation mark' appearance).

28. D ★★

This is a patch of scarring alopecia. Scarring alopecia can be caused by trauma, radiation, lichen planopilaris, and discoid lupus erythematosus. Atrophic plaques over the face or ears are characteristic of discoid lupus.

29. G ★★

This is the typical 'moth-eaten' appearance of tinea capitis. It would require treatment with a systemic antifungal agent, such as griseofulvin or terbinafine.

30. B ★★

This is alopecia areata universalis (loss of all body hair).

General feedback on 25–30: OHCS 9th edn → pp. 598, 602

Chapter 8

Anaesthesia and intensive care

Alex Bonner and James Dawson

Anaesthesia is a relatively young specialty by comparison with its counterparts. William Morton administered the first anaesthetic in 1846 in Boston, Massachusetts. The Royal College of Anaesthetists was created from the Royal College of Surgeons in 1948, and anaesthetists now form the largest group of hospital-based doctors.

Anaesthetists are highly trained physicians whose role is by no means limited to the operating theatre. They oversee the patient journey through the peri-operative period (which involves optimization of the sick patient prior to surgery), ensuring the safe induction of, maintenance of, and emergence from anaesthesia, as well as the care of the patient in the early post-operative period. Anaesthetic skills are also requested during management of the critically ill in the Emergency Department, and during the care of the parturient mother, in providing analgesic, anaesthetic, and intensive care input. Anaesthetists have an important role in the practice of intensive care, where complementary experience in medicine is useful. Other roles of the anaesthetist include provision of acute and chronic pain services. Other subspecialty interests include regional, paediatric, cardiothoracic, and neuroanaesthesia.

Anaesthesia is a highly practical specialty, with a strong emphasis on the basic sciences underpinning its practice. Physiology and pharmacology exert their effects with immediacy. Therefore an affinity for these disciplines is desirable. Anaesthetists need to be able to assimilate knowledge of the basic sciences with skills in history and examination, in order to plan for and respond to patient needs. In answering these questions, you will be asked to use similar skills.

Alex Bonner

QUESTIONS

Single Best Answers

1. A 70-year-old man has had worsening shortness of breath for 2 days. He has a 50-pack-year history of cigarette smoking, but otherwise has no previous medical history. He appears unwell, with a reduced level of consciousness and inadequate respiratory effort. The following arterial blood gas levels are obtained while he is breathing through a facemask with a reservoir bag, with an oxygen flow rate of 15 L/minute:

- pH 7.14
- pO_2 10.1 kPa
- pCO_2 9.8 kPa
- bicarbonate 29.2 mmol/L
- base excess +9.4.

Which is the single best description of the acid–base derangement? ★

A Metabolic acidosis with respiratory compensation

B Metabolic alkalosis with respiratory compensation

C Mixed respiratory and metabolic acidosis

D Respiratory acidosis with evidence of metabolic compensation

E Respiratory acidosis with no evidence of metabolic compensation

2. A 19-year-old man fractured his right lower leg about 30 minutes ago, while playing football. He was carried off the pitch on a stretcher. He is in discomfort and there is some bloodstaining on his sock. His right lower leg is immobilized in a box splint. He has an open fracture of his right distal tibia. There is no distal neurovascular deficit and he is haemodynamically stable; blood loss is estimated to be minimal. He has no other injuries and is fully alert. Which is the single most appropriate initial analgesia to give? ★

A IM diclofenac

B IV alfentanil

C IV morphine

D IV paracetamol

E Oral codeine phosphate

3. A 19-year-old woman is brought into the Emergency Department by paramedics. She was found unconscious in her bed by her parents, who also found empty packets of several prescription medications and a bottle of vodka. She does not open her eyes at all but withdraws to pain. She makes no verbal response. Which is her single Glasgow Coma Scale score? ★

A 3

B 6

C 9

D 12

E 15

4. A 56-year-old man was thrombolysed for an anterior myocardial infarction 6 hours ago. His pain had eased, but then he suddenly had severe central crushing chest pain radiating into his left arm. He is now unconscious with no signs of life. The defibrillator is attached and the monitor displays the rhythm shown in Plate 8.1 (see Colour Plate section). Cardiopulmonary resuscitation (CPR) with chest compressions and bag-valve-mask ventilation is started. He has IV access. Which is the single next most appropriate management? ★

A Continue CPR for 2 minutes

B Defibrillation

C Endotracheal intubation

D IV atropine

E IV epinephrine (adrenaline)

5. A 24-year-old woman is having a simple surgical procedure under an upper limb nerve block. Shortly after the surgeon commences the procedure, she feels light-headed and dizzy. She experiences ringing in her ears and tingling around her mouth. Which is the single most likely diagnosis? ★

A Acute labyrinthitis

B Anaphylaxis

C Failure of anaesthetic

D Local anaesthetic toxicity

E Vasovagal attack

6. A 34-year-old woman has been admitted to hospital with cellulitis of her forearm. She has just been given her second dose of IV penicillin. She now has chest tightness, difficulty in breathing, and feels dizzy. She has a diffuse urticarial rash all over her body, and bilateral expiratory and inspiratory wheeze. Her pulse rate is 120 bpm, her blood pressure is 80/40 mmHg, and her oxygen saturation is 91% on room air. Which is the single most appropriate initial management? ★

A IM epinephrine (adrenaline) 0.5 mg

B IV chlorphenamine 10 mg

C IV epinephrine (adrenaline) 1 mg

D IV hydrocortisone 100 mg

E Take blood for serum mast cell tryptase

7. A 76-year-old woman had a left total knee replacement 4 days ago. She is normally fit and healthy. She has had an uncomplicated postoperative recovery, but recent observations give her a Modified Early Warning Score of 6, whereas 1 hour ago the score was 2. Her pulse rate is 120 bpm, her blood pressure is 90/45 mmHg, her oxygen saturation is 90% on room air, her respiratory rate is 30 breaths/minute, and her temperature is 37.5°C. She is alert but has chest pain and shortness of breath. Which is the single most likely cause of her acute deterioration? ★

A Cardiac tamponade

B Myocardial infarction

C Pneumonia

D Pneumothorax

E Pulmonary embolism

8. A 24-year-old woman is 32 weeks pregnant with her first child. She has had pregnancy-induced hypertension. Her booking blood pressure was 125/76 mmHg. She has come to the labour suite with a headache and she has some ankle oedema. Her blood pressure is now 145/92 mmHg, and urinalysis shows 3+ proteinuria. She suddenly loses consciousness and has a tonic–clonic seizure. She is put in the recovery position and given supplementary oxygen. Which is the single most appropriate treatment? ★

A IV lorazepam

B IV magnesium sulphate

C IV phenytoin

D Oral methyldopa

E Sublingual nifedipine

9. A 19-year-old man has had a recurrent dislocation of his left shoulder. He has been given 20 mg of IV midazolam and his shoulder is now reduced. He is now unconscious and has stopped breathing. Which is the single most appropriate immediate management? ★

A Connect ECG monitoring

B Give IV flumazenil

C Give IV naloxone

D Intubate the patient

E Open the airway with a jaw thrust

10. A 63-year-old woman had a redo total hip replacement under general anaesthetic 3 days ago. She now has chest pain, which developed suddenly and is worse on inspiration. Her pulse rate is 110 bpm, her oxygen saturation is 90% on 5 L of oxygen by mask, and her temperature is 37.4°C. Which single investigation is likely to confirm the diagnosis? ★

A Chest X-ray

B CT pulmonary angiogram

C ECG

D Echocardiography

E Cardiac enzymes

11. A 64-year-old woman had an inferior myocardial infarction (MI) 12 hours ago, and has been successfully thrombolysed. She suddenly develops a profound narrow complex bradycardia with a rate of 30 bpm. Her blood pressure is 75/39 mmHg and she feels dizzy and sick. Which is the single most appropriate immediate management? ★

A IV amiodarone

B IV atropine

C IV isoprenaline

D Transcutaneous (external) cardiac pacing

E Transvenous cardiac pacing

12. A 6-week-old boy, who was born prematurely, has had vomiting and lethargy for 5 days. He has sunken eyes and reduced skin turgor. His capillary refill time is 4 seconds. The following arterial blood gas sample is obtained:

- pH 7.52
- P_aCO_2 5.0 kPa
- P_aO_2 11.0 kPa
- HCO_3 34.2 mmol/L
- base excess +9.1.

Which is the single best description of his metabolic status? ★

A Metabolic acidosis without respiratory compensation

B Metabolic alkalosis with respiratory compensation

C Metabolic alkalosis without respiratory compensation

D Respiratory alkalosis with metabolic compensation

E Respiratory alkalosis without metabolic compensation

13. A 68-year-old man has chronic obstructive pulmonary disease (COPD). He has been involved in a motor vehicle collision, and has a fractured femur and signs of a tension pneumothorax. His oxygen saturation is 76% on room air. He is being prepared for a needle thoracocentesis. Which is the single most appropriate means of oxygen delivery to use? ★

A Face-mask continuous positive airway pressure (CPAP)

B Immediate intubation and ventilation

C Nasal cannulae

D Non-rebreather mask with reservoir bag

E Venturi mask with 35% oxygen delivery

14. A 20-year-old man is undergoing his first ever general anaesthetic for an elective tonsillectomy. Shortly after administration of the induction agents, he becomes unwell. Which is the single most likely first sign indicating that he may be having an anaphylactic reaction? ★

A Angio-oedema

B Cough

C Desaturation

D Hypotension

E Rash

15. A 55-year-old woman with a history of chronic pain presents to the Emergency Department with morning somnolence, blurred vision, and urinary retention. She states that her general practitioner has recently started a new chronic pain medication, but she cannot remember the name of the drug. Which single drug, used in the treatment of chronic pain, is most likely to cause this group of side-effects? ★ ★

A Amitriptyline

B Carbamazepine

C Gabapentin

D Morphine

E Sodium valproate

16. A 35-year-old man is seen on the day-case unit prior to an arthroscopy for knee pain. He describes himself as 'fit and well', and does not smoke. He takes inhalers for asthma, which is well controlled, and has no other medical problems. Which single American Society of Anesthesiologists (ASA) grade best describes his physical status? ★ ★

A I

B II

C III

D IV

E V

17. A 31-year-old woman is scheduled for an elective laparoscopic cholecystectomy. After intubation, the CO_2 (capnography) trace diminishes, she begins to desaturate, and the anaesthetist is unable to hear air entry when auscultating over the chest, despite being able to hand ventilate her easily. Which is the single most likely cause for this? ★ ★

A Anaphylaxis

B Cardiac arrest

C Monitoring failure

D Oesophageal intubation

E Bilateral pneumothoraces

18. Urgent help is required in the anaesthetic room. A patient has become rapidly unwell during induction of anaesthesia. He has generalized muscle rigidity and tachycardia, and appears sweaty. His blood pressure is normal. Which is the single most likely diagnosis? ★ ★

A Acute dystonia

B Anaphylaxis

C Epileptic seizure

D Malignant hyperthermia

E Suxamethonium apnoea

19. A 49-year-old woman has presumed sepsis arising from her biliary tract. She is known to have hypertension and gallstones. The admitting team have obtained IV access and taken blood. The woman has also received a dose of broad-spectrum antibiotics. Her blood pressure is 91/40 mmHg and her serum lactate level is 3.6 mmol/L. Which is the single most important next management step, according to the Surviving Sepsis Campaign (2008)? ★ ★

A Commence a vasopressor infusion

B Give a minimum 20 mL/kg fluid bolus

C Insert a peripheral arterial line

D Insert a central venous catheter

E Recheck the serum lactate level

20. A new mother on the obstetric ward had a forceps delivery under epidural anaesthesia 2 days ago. She initially made a good recovery and was walking on the ward. However, she now has back pain, leg weakness, and bladder dysfunction. She has lower limb motor and sensory dysfunction on testing. Which is the single most likely diagnosis? ★ ★

A Bacterial meningitis

B Brown-Séquard syndrome

C Epidural haematoma

D Peroneal nerve palsy

E Prolapsed intervertebral disc

21. A previously fit and well 34-year-old man is undergoing surgery for a fractured right femur. He is under a general anaesthetic and the orthopaedic surgeons have just inserted the femoral nail. Intra-operative blood loss is estimated to be about 2000 mL. He has been given 3000 mL of IV fluid throughout the operation. A bedside haemoglobin test gives a haemoglobin level of 6.9 g/dL. His pulse rate is 100 bpm and his blood pressure is 125/75 mmHg. No further blood loss is anticipated. Which is the single most appropriate next step in management? ★ ★

A Administration of recombinant activated factor VIIa

B Prescribing post-operative iron tablets

C Transfusion of fully cross-matched blood

D Transfusion of group O rhesus-negative blood

E Transfusion of group-specific blood

22. A 53-year-old woman returns to the recovery room after a laparoscopic cholecystectomy. The procedure was technically difficult and lasted longer than anticipated. Her temperature in recovery is 32.9°C. Which single physical process accounts for the greatest heat loss intra-operatively? ★ ★

A Conduction

B Convection

C Humidification

D Radiation

E Respiration

23. A 31-year-old man has sustained a cut to his right (dominant) hand while at work. The cut is on the palm of the hand on the radial aspect. A median nerve block at the wrist is planned to provide sufficient anaesthesia for the wound to be explored and sutured. Which single option describes where the median nerve lies at the wrist? ★ ★

A Between the tendons of the palmaris longus and the flexor pollicis longus

B Lateral to the radial artery

C Medial to the ulnar artery

D Medial to the ulnar nerve

E Superficial to the flexor retinaculum

24. A 17-year-old man has HbAS (sickle cell trait). He is undergoing repair of a fractured radius under general anaesthetic. During the procedure, the surgeon uses a tourniquet to create a bloodless field, and K-wires the fracture. The patient receives IV fluids, analgesia, and post-operatively is given oxygen. Which single factor is associated with an increased risk of sickle cell crisis? ★ ★

A IV fluid therapy

B Opioid analgesia

C Oxygen therapy

D Prophylactic antibiotics

E Tourniquet use

25. An 82-year-old man has had a transurethral resection of the prostate (TURP) procedure under spinal anaesthetic. The procedure was long and the surgeon required large volumes of irrigating fluid. In recovery, the patient becomes increasingly agitated and confused, his Glasgow Coma Scale score falls, and he requires intubation. Which is the single most likely metabolic abnormality to account for this? ★ ★

A Hyperglycaemia

B Hypernatraemia

C Hypoglycaemia

D Hypokalaemia

E Hyponatraemia

26. A 6-year-old child weighing approximately 20 kg is brought into the Emergency Department. She has sustained burns to the torso covering an estimated 20% of body surface area (BSA). The child is haemodynamically stable. Which is the single correct volume of fluid to administer in the first 8 hours following admission? ★ ★ ★

A 250 mL

B 400 mL

C 600 mL

D 800 mL

E 1000 mL

27. A 42-year-old woman had a partial thyroidectomy 24 hours ago. Her pre-operative haemoglobin level was 11.4 g/dL. Today's result is 3.8 g/dL. She is pain free, her pulse rate is 85 bpm, and her blood pressure is 118/76 mmHg. Blood loss was estimated to be about 300 mL, and there is minimal fluid in the surgical drain. Her neck is not distended and the wound site is clean and dry. Which is the single most likely cause of the anaemia? ★ ★ ★

A Bone-marrow failure

B Iron deficiency

C Major intra-operative haemorrhage

D Ongoing post-operative haemorrhage

E Spurious result

28. A 29-year-old man has been on the Intensive Therapy Unit for 2 days following a serious motor vehicle collision. He is making no respiratory effort, and tests show that he has brainstem death. The medical team is planning to talk to the relatives about the possibility of organ donation. Which single advice is correct in relation to organ donation? ★ ★ ★ ★

A Organs can only be harvested once the donor's heart has stopped beating

B Organ donation can only take place if the donor is on the organ donor register or carried an organ donation card

C Organs of patients who are human immunodeficiency virus (HIV) positive are usually taken

D Organs will usually be harvested if the donor is on the organ donation register, even if the next of kin do not wish for organs to be donated

E The next of kin can specify if they do not want particular organs to be donated

29. A 35-year-old woman is undergoing a diagnostic laparoscopy for pelvic pain. She is deemed to be at high risk for post-operative nausea and vomiting. Which single class of drugs can be used in the prophylaxis of post-operative nausea and vomiting? ★ ★ ★ ★

A Anticonvulsants

B Benzodiazepines

C Corticosteroids

D Opioids

E Smooth muscle relaxants

30. An 80-year-old woman is undergoing palliative care for inoperable cancer. She has copious secretions in the upper airway that are troublesome, and is requesting something to relieve this symptom. Which single group of drugs is the most appropriate to prescribe? ★ ★ ★ ★

A Acetylcholinesterase inhibitors

B Anticholinergic agents

C Antihistamines

D Dopamine antagonists

E Sympathomimetic agents

Extended Matching Questions

Causes of poisoning

For each patient, choose the *single* most likely diagnosis from the list of options below. Each option may be used once, more than once, or not at all. ★

A Alcohol poisoning

B Amitriptyline overdose

C Benzodiazepine overdose

D Beta-blocker overdose

E Carbamazepine overdose

F Carbon monoxide poisoning

G Digoxin toxicity

H Lithium overdose

I Opioid overdose

J Oxygen toxicity

K Paracetamol overdose

L Paraquat poisoning

1. A young man has been found unresponsive on a street corner. His airway is being maintained with an oropharyngeal airway device and a jaw thrust, and his breathing is infrequent and shallow. He has pinpoint pupils. His pulse rate is 70 bpm, his blood pressure is 90/50 mmHg, and his Glasgow Coma Scale score is 3/15.

2. A 19-year-old woman has abdominal pain and vomiting. She took an overdose of tablets two nights ago while drunk, but is not sure what the tablets were. She has right upper quadrant tenderness. Her pulse rate is 100 bpm, her blood pressure is 102/59 mmHg, and her Glasgow Coma Scale score is 15/15. Blood tests show:

- bilirubin 100 μmol/L
- alanine aminotransferase 780 IU/L
- international normalized ratio (INR) 5.0.

3. A 21-year-old woman has taken an overdose of her mother's prescription tablets. She is pale and clammy. Her pulse rate is 30 bpm and her blood pressure is 75/33 mmHg. An ECG shows a profound sinus bradycardia.

4. A 59-year-old man has been found in his car in a remote location by the police. He was initially unresponsive. In the Emergency Department he is drowsy and confused. He is very pink in colour. His pulse rate is 90 bpm, his blood pressure is 110/50 mmHg, and his oxygen saturation on finger probe is 100% on high-flow oxygen.

5. A 78-year-old man has mistakenly taken too many of his regular tablets. He is vomiting and mildly confused, and he says that everything looks yellow. His pulse rate is 40 bpm and his blood pressure is 90/43 mmHg. An ECG shows very slow atrial fibrillation.

Drugs used in emergencies

For each patient, choose the *single* most appropriate initial management from the list of options below. Each option may be used once, more than once, or not at all. ★ ★ ★

A Adenosine 3 mg IV

B Amiodarone 150 mg IV

C Atropine 2–3 mg IV

D Calcium gluconate 10% 10 mL IV

E Calcium resonium 30 g per rectum

F Chlorpheniramine 10 mg IV

G Diazepam 30 mg per rectum

H Epinephrine (adrenaline) 0.5 mg IV

I Epinephrine 0.5 mg IM

J Epinephrine 1 mg IV

K Epinephrine 1 mg IM

L Glucagon 1 mg IV

M Hydrocortisone 200 mg IV

N Lorazepam 4 mg IV

O Magnesium sulphate 1.2–2 g IV

P Naloxone 400 micrograms

Q Potassium chloride 20 mmol

R Prednisolone 30 mg orally

S Salbutamol 3–20 mg/minute IV infusion

T Salbutamol 5 mg nebulized

U Sodium bicarbonate 8.4% 50 mL IV

6. A 66-year-old man who was recently discharged from hospital following a myocardial infarction presents with chest pain. His ECG shows a broad complex tachycardia at a rate of 150 bpm. He has failed to respond to synchronized DC cardioversion.

7. A 24-year-old man has had a severe reaction to peanuts. He is cyanotic, wheezy, and covered in an urticarial rash. His blood pressure is 85/60 mmHg.

8. A 30-year-old man with asthma has a peak expiratory flow rate of less than 33% predicted. His respiratory rate is 26 breaths/minute and his pulse rate is 115 bpm. Oxygen is given at 15 L/minute via a face mask with a reservoir bag.

9. A 45-year-old man has had profuse watery diarrhoea and vomiting for 5 days. He has not been able to tolerate oral fluids and is profoundly dehydrated. While the results of his blood tests are awaited, an ECG is performed, which shows tall tented T waves, flattening of P waves, and widening of the QRS complexes.

10. A 61-year-old man with a history of depression and self-harm is brought into the Emergency Department. He has ingested a large volume of commercial pesticide. He is wheezy and has excessive salivation and lacrimation. He also has diarrhoea and his pupils are meiotic. His heart rate is 60 bpm.

ANSWERS

Single Best Answers

1. D ★

The blood gas shows a marked respiratory acidosis. As is common in patients with smoking-related lung disease, a degree of metabolic compensation for a chronically elevated pCO_2 occurs, shown by the raised bicarbonate level. However, this man is unwell with a grossly elevated pCO_2, which exceeds the buffering capacity of the blood. He has a reduced level of consciousness from carbon dioxide narcosis.

The flow chart below sets out a step-by-step guide on how to approach blood gases:

Acidosis: pH 7.35	Alkalosis: pH 7.45
Look at the base excess first: Normal (–3 to +3) = respiratory acidosis, and pCO_2 will be raised (> 6 kPa)	Look at the base excess first: Normal (–3 to +3) = respiratory alkalosis, and pCO_2 will be low (< 4.5 kPa)
High negative (> –4) = metabolic acidosis. If pCO_2 is normal (4.5–6 kPa), it is just a metabolic acidosis. If pCO_2 is low (< 4.5 kPa), there is respiratory compensation. If the pCO_2 is also high, it is a mixed acidosis	High positive (> +4) = metabolic alkalosis. If pCO_2 is normal (4.5–6 kPa), it is just a metabolic alkalosis. If pCO_2 is high (> 6 kPa), there is respiratory compensation. If pCO_2 is low, it is a mixed alkalosis
High positive (> +4) = respiratory acidosis with renal compensation. The pCO_2 will be high (> 6 kPa)	High negative (> –4) = respiratory alkalosis with renal compensation. The pCO_2 will be low (< 4.5 kPa)

2. C ★   OHCS 9th edn → p. 636

Acute severe pain is best managed with strong opioids, such as morphine. Common routes of administration of the strong opioids in acute pain include the intravenous, intramuscular, oral, intranasal, and subcutaneous routes. Intravenous administration will provide the most rapid pain relief, and avoids first-pass metabolism by the liver (first-pass metabolism mainly affects orally administered drugs). The strong opioids should be titrated to effect. The intramuscular route is useful in a ward setting, but perfusion to peripheral muscles can be impaired due to the sympathetic activity that follows acute injury. This results in delayed onset of action, with potentially late onset of side-effects once perfusion to muscle is restored, and would be less suitable in this setting. Alfentanil is a very short-acting opioid that is usually only used in the operating theatre.

The World Health Organization (WHO) analgesic ladder offers a stepwise approach to pain management, although the severity of acute pain needs to be assessed to ensure that treatment begins on the appropriate 'rung' of the ladder.

Treatment of this patient with paracetamol or a weak opioid alone would be insufficient to control his acute pain. Combining a strong opioid with paracetamol and a non-steroidal anti-inflammatory drug (e.g. diclofenac or ibuprofen) will reduce the overall amount of opioid that is needed to control his pain. This is beneficial, as it will minimize the risk of opioid side-effects (sedation, nausea and vomiting, constipation, etc.).

→ www.ganfyd.org/images/thumb/7/77/WHO_Analgesic_Ladder. png/550px-WHO_Analgesic_Ladder.png

3. B ★   OHCS 9th edn → p. 720

The Glasgow Coma Scale (GCS) is used to assess and record the level of consciousness of a patient. Although it was developed for use on traumatized patients, the GCS is used to assess virtually all patients who present with a depressed level of consciousness, irrespective of the cause.

Best eye response	Score
No eye opening	1
Eyes open to pain	2
Eyes open to command	3
Eyes open spontaneously	4
Best motor response	
No motor response	1
Extensor posturing to pain	2
Abnormal flexor posturing to pain	3
Withdraws to pain (normal flexion)	4
Localizing response to pain	5
Obeys command	6
Best verbal response	
No sounds	1
Incomprehensible sound	2
Inappropriate speech	3
Confused conversation	4
Normal	5

4. B ★

This man has ventricular fibrillation (VF) and requires immediate electrical defibrillation. The fibrillating heart has electrical activity, but this is uncoordinated and so the heart cannot function as a pump. Passing electricity through the heart (defibrillation) causes transient cessation of all endogenous electrical activity. Once this occurs, the intrinsic pacemakers should take over and result in coordinated contractions of the atria and ventricles being resumed.

Chest compressions alone are very unlikely to cardiovert VF into a perfusing rhythm, and if a defibrillator is immediately available, a defibrillating shock should be given as soon as VF is identified. Once VF has been identified, the initial shock takes precedence over airway, breathing, and the administration of any drugs.

The stepwise management of VF and pulseless ventricular tachycardia (VT) are the same, and are outlined in the Adult Advanced Life Support Algorithm.

→ www.resus.org.uk/pages/alsalgo.pdf

5. D ★   OHCS 9th edn → p. 632

Whenever local anaesthetic is used, the possibility of toxicity should be considered. The first symptoms of local anaesthetic toxicity are due to central nervous system (CNS) stimulation (tinnitus, circumoral paraesthesia, light-headedness, and dizziness), followed by CNS depression and cardiovascular collapse. Injection of local anaesthetic should always follow careful aspiration to ensure that the needle is not in a blood vessel. If a patient complains of symptoms suggestive of toxicity, the operator should immediately stop injecting anaesthetic. The management of local anaesthetic toxicity can be aided by the administration of intralipid.

→ www.aagbi.org/sites/default/files/la_toxicity_2010_0.pdf

6. A ★

This patient is having an anaphylactic reaction, probably to the administered antibiotics. The priorities in management should follow the Airway, Breathing, Circulation approach (see the Adult Advanced Life Support Algorithm).

If anaphylaxis is suspected, the precipitant should be stopped (e.g. stop antibiotic infusion) and the patient given IM epinephrine 0.5 mg (0.5 mL of 1:1000 epinephrine). It is unlikely that IM epinephrine will cause an adverse event if it later transpires that the patient was not having an anaphylactic reaction. If in doubt, the IM epinephrine should be given.

Chlorphenamine, hydrocortisone, and taking blood for mast cell tryptase are all indicated in cases of anaphylaxis, but epinephrine takes priority. Common precipitants of anaphylaxis include blood products, colloid fluids, antibiotics, and muscle relaxants.

→ www.resus.org.uk/pages/anaalgo.pdf

7. E ★

This woman has had lower-limb surgery and is likely to have been fairly immobile for the last 4 days. She is at high risk of a deep vein thrombosis and subsequent pulmonary embolism. This is the most likely pathology.

Beck's triad (muffled heart sounds, raised jugular venous pressure, and hypotension) would make cardiac tamponade more likely, but this is not pathognomonic. Equally, there is no history of ischaemic heart disease, and an acute myocardial infarction is unlikely to give rise to desaturation unless there has been gross heart failure. Pneumonia is relatively common in the post-operative population, but usually has a more gradual onset of cough, pyrexia, anorexia, and lethargy. Pneumothoraces can be rapid in onset, but again there is no reason (e.g. pre-existing lung disease, positive pressure ventilation, central lines, etc.) to suggest that this patient is at risk from these.

The Modified Early Warning Score (MEWS) is an objective way of highlighting adverse patient physiology so that appropriate help can be sought:

Total score	Action
2	Repeat observations in 30 minutes
3	Inform a junior doctor
> 4	Request a junior doctor immediately

The MEWS is calculated as follows:

	3	2	1	0	1	2	3
Respiratory rate (breaths/ minute)		< 9		9–14	15–20	21–29	≥ 30
Heart rate (bpm)		< 40	41–50	51–100	101–110	111–129	≥ 130
Systolic blood pressure (mmHg)	< 70	71–80	81–100	101–199		≥ 200	
Temperature (°C)		< 35		35–38.4		≥ 38.5	
AVPU				Alert	Reacts to Voice	Reacts to Pain	Unresponsive

→ www.gp-training.net/protocol/cardiovascular/dvt.htm

→ http://qjmed.oxfordjournals.org/cgi/content/full/94/10/521

8. B ★

This patient initially had pre-eclampsia. This condition is diagnosed after 20 weeks' gestation when there is hypertension (systolic blood pressure greater than 140 mmHg and/or diastolic blood pressure greater than 90 mmHg) or a rise in systolic blood pressure of more than 30 mmHg or a rise in diastolic blood pressure of more than 15 mmHg compared with the booking blood pressure, and greater than 300 mg/dL per 24 hours of protein in the urine (in practical terms, more than 2+ on urinalysis). Eclampsia is diagnosed when a patient with pre-eclampsia has a seizure. The Magpie Trial demonstrated that patients with pre-eclampsia were less likely to go on to develop eclampsia if they were given IV magnesium. This and other work has also formed the basis of the first-line treatment of eclampsia with IV magnesium.

The Magpie Trial Collaborative Group (2002). Do women with pre-eclampsia, and their babies, benefit from magnesium sulphate? The Magpie Trial: a randomized placebo-controlled trial. *Lancet* **360**: 1331–1332.

→ http://emedicine.medscape.com/article/261435-overview

9. E ★

This patient has respiratory depression secondary to benzodiazepine excess. The immediate approach to any critically ill patient begins with airway assessment and management if indicated. This must take place before moving on to breathing and then to circulation, as outlined in the Adult Advanced Life Support Algorithm (ALS). If the patient's airway is not patent or safe after a jaw thrust and use of airway adjuncts (e.g. Guedel airway), they may need intubation. Applying ECG leads is part of the assessment of the circulation.

Naloxone is the reversal agent used in opioid overdose. Flumazenil is the reversal agent used in benzodiazepine overdose, but again airway management takes precedence over flumazenil in this case.

→ www.resus.org.uk/pages/als.pdf

10. B ★

This history points towards the diagnosis of pulmonary embolism in the post-operative period. Pelvic surgery and orthopaedic surgery are risk factors for pulmonary embolism. Although chest X-ray and ECG may point towards pulmonary embolism, in most hospitals the 'gold standard' investigation for confirming the diagnosis is CT pulmonary angiography.

11. B ★

This patient has a bradycardia, which is probably secondary to her inferior MI, and which is causing cardiovascular compromise (hypotension). In accordance with the Adult Bradycardia Algorithm, she has adverse signs of her bradycardia, and the first-line treatment should be with IV atropine (an anticholinergic drug). If the bradycardia persists, IV isoprenaline (a β-adrenoceptor agonist) and transcutaneous (external) and transvenous cardiac pacing may all be utilized.

Amiodarone is used to treat tachyarrhythmias, and often results in bradycardia.

→ www.resus.org.uk/pages/bradalgo.pdf

12. C ★   OHCS 9th edn → p. 172

A child with pyloric stenosis classically presents with a metabolic alkalosis due to loss of acid from the upper gastrointestinal tract. A flow chart giving a step-by-step guide on how to approach blood gases in shown in Single Best Answer 1.

13. D ★

This man's tension pneumothorax is life-threatening. He also needs a high concentration of oxygen to be delivered to his functioning lung, as he is grossly hypoxaemic. Some colleagues may voice concern that a patient with COPD potentially has a 'hypoxic drive', and that giving oxygen will cause the patient to hypoventilate, retain carbon dioxide, and become drowsy. This is not a concern in this life-threatening emergency setting—the patient is likely to die of hypoxaemia or circulatory collapse secondary to the tension pneumothorax first, unless he is treated. The oxygen concentration can be reduced once the patient is more stable.

A face mask with a non-rebreather valve and reservoir bag will deliver about 80% oxygen when the oxygen is turned on to 15 L/minute. Nasal cannulae will deliver about 28%, and the Venturi system will deliver 35%, both of which are insufficient in this setting. Face-mask CPAP is likely to expand this pneumothorax further, as would intubation and ventilation. A chest drain must be sited before commencing either of these in this situation.

14. D ★   OHCS 9th edn → p. 237

Hypotension is observed more commonly than any other clinical sign in patients who are developing anaphylactic reactions. Any of the other signs mentioned may still occur.

→ www.aagbi.org/sites/default/files/anaphylaxis_2009_0.pdf

15. A ★★

Amitriptyline is a tricyclic antidepressant, but it is also used in the treatment of neuropathic pain. This class of drugs has an analgesic effect that is independent of any antidepressant effect. The drug blocks many neurotransmitters in the central nervous system, including norepinephrine and serotonin, but it is the anticholinergic actions that would cause the side-effects described here. Drugs that antagonize acetylcholine at cholinergic receptors (e.g. atropine and hyoscine) often cause these effects.

The other drugs are all used in the treatment of chronic pain. All of these agents have significant side-effects. Titrating drugs to achieve the right balance between the desired effect and tolerable side-effects is paramount in this setting. Warning patients about what side-effects to expect and how to manage them is an important aspect of drug prescribing. For example, morning somnolence (tiredness) may be overcome by taking the evening dose 1 or 2 hours earlier.

16. B ★★   OHCS 9th edn → p. 615

Class II refers to a patient with a mild systemic disease. The ASA grading of patient status was introduced in the 1960s. Although simple, it has been shown to correlate with the risks associated with anaesthesia and surgery, and therefore forms part of the pre-operative assessment of all patients undergoing general anaesthesia.

ASA grade	Description	Mortality rate (%)
I	Normally healthy individual	0.1
II	Patient with mild systemic disease	0.2
III	Patient with severe systemic disease that is not incapacitating	1.8
IV	Patient with incapacitating systemic disease that is a constant threat to life	7.8
V	Moribund patient who is not expected to survive for 24 hours with or without an operation	9.4

The mortality rates quoted above are an average for both elective and emergency surgery. The suffix E is added to denote an emergency operation.

17. D ★★   OHCS 9th edn → p. 627

Anaphylaxis usually presents with a combination of bronchospasm, rash, tachycardia, and hypotension. As the patient is easy to hand ventilate, anaphylaxis is unlikely, as bronchospastic lungs require high airway pressures.

Cardiac arrest would cause an absent pulse oximetry trace, and breath sounds would still be audible while the patient was being hand ventilated.

A failure of monitoring equipment is unlikely to give this picture, as both the capnography and the pulse oximetry modules would have to be faulty at the same time, and the patient might well become cyanotic.

The occurrence of bilateral pneumothoraces would be very unlucky, but could give rise to this situation. However, probability dictates that this is very unlikely.

Oesophageal intubation is the most likely cause here, and could be confirmed by auscultating over the stomach and hearing air entry when hand ventilating the patient. Its management involves removal of the misplaced tube, re-oxygenating the patient with mask ventilation, and then intubating the trachea.

18. D ★ ★   OHCS 9th edn → p. 628

Malignant hyperthermia is an inherited disorder of calcium metabolism that affects skeletal muscle. It is most often triggered by suxamethonium or the volatile anaesthetic agents. Its presentation varies from one individual to another, but it should be considered when there is unexplained tachycardia, especially in the presence of tachypnoea, muscle rigidity, or an increase in end-tidal pCO_2. Malignant hyperthermia can be a life-threatening condition, or it may present more insidiously. Emergency management includes removal of the trigger agent, cooling, and treatment with dantrolene (a drug that interferes with skeletal muscle contraction). Without treatment, the mortality rate is approximately 75%; with treatment, mortality is significantly reduced.

None of the other diagnoses classically present as described here. Acute dystonia is often triggered by neuroleptic agents, and typically presents in the first few days of new treatment. It is rarely associated with anaesthesia. Suxamethonium apnoea is an inherited deficiency of plasma cholinesterase, resulting in delayed metabolism of suxamethonium and therefore prolongation of neuromuscular blockade.

19. B ★ ★

Vasoactive mediators from the infective agent and from damaged endothelium are causing widespread vasodilatation, hypotension, and a resultant tachycardia. The first goal of the management of septic shock is to ensure adequate filling (pre-load), as measured by the central venous pressure (CVP). Once the patient is adequately filled, if hypotension and shock persist, a vasopressor should then be commenced, such as noradrenaline (norepinephrine, which acts predominantly upon α_1-adrenoceptors).

A central line will allow the CVP to be measured, but more important than the specific value recorded is the trend in pressure in response to fluid boluses. If the CVP continues to rise, this usually suggests that more fluid is needed, whereas a plateau in the CVP suggests that adequate filling has been achieved. A central line will also allow some drugs to be administered that would otherwise be irritant to smaller peripheral veins.

An arterial line will be useful in the High-Dependency Unit/Intensive Therapy Unit setting, but is not a priority in the first instance. Similarly, rechecking the serum lactate level is unlikely to be of use within the first 6 hours.

20. C ★★

The history points to a rare but very serious complication of epidural anaesthesia. A haematoma that is formed following insertion of a catheter into the epidural space can expand and cause neurological compromise. Traumatic insertion or derangements of clotting increase the likelihood of haematoma formation.

21. C ★★

Loss of more than 20% of the circulating volume is regarded as a significant blood loss, and in most circumstances this needs to be replaced with a blood transfusion. Circulating volume is approximately 70 mL/kg, so it is around 4900 mL in a 70 kg man. In this case there is time to obtain fully cross-matched blood, which usually takes about 45 minutes to become available. This blood will be thoroughly matched for the patient's blood group (A, B, AB, or O), rhesus D status (negative or positive), and for the rarer antibodies/antigens. Type-specific blood takes about 20 minutes to become available, and is matched for blood group and rhesus D status, but not for the rarer antibodies/antigens. Group O rhesus-negative blood (universal donor blood) should be available immediately in most clinical areas, but carries the risk of the patient raising antibodies to the rarer antigens, which can cause problems with future blood transfusions. The decision as to which blood to request will depend upon the level of clinical urgency.

The following link is to the National Blood Service website, and shows the current stocks of blood:

→ www.blood.co.uk/StockGraph/stocklevelstandard.aspx

22. D ★★   OHCS 9th edn → p. 628

Radiation accounts for approximately 40% of the heat lost from the body. In addition, convection (30%), respiration (including humidification) (20%), and conduction (10%) are all important, and their relative contributions vary depending on the environment. Space blankets are designed to reduce heat loss from radiation.

23. **A** ★★   OHCS 9th edn → p. 761

The median nerve lies between the two prominent tendons at the wrist (the palmaris longus and flexor pollicis longus), and is deep to the flexor retinaculum within the carpal tunnel. Swelling within the carpal tunnel gives rise to 'carpal tunnel syndrome', which is caused by compression upon the median nerve.

The ulna bone, ulnar nerve, and ulnar artery are medial to the median nerve, and the radial artery lies lateral to it.

24. **E** ★★

Use of a tourniquet is associated with precipitation of sickle cell crisis. If a tourniquet must be used, the limb should be thoroughly exsanguinated prior to inflation. All of the other options are associated with minimization of the risk of a crisis, and should form part of the peri-operative care where appropriate.

25. **E** ★★

TURP syndrome is a complication of TURP, and is caused by the combination of fluid overload and hyponatraemia, which results from high volumes of hypotonic irrigating fluid being used over the open prostate gland. It can be complicated by hyperglycinaemia (not hyperglycaemia) as a result of the glycine irrigation fluid that is used by the surgeons. Therefore the mental state of these patients should be regularly assessed peri-operatively, and any sign of confusion should be a cause for concern. Long procedures are a risk factor for TURP syndrome. Management consists of slow correction of the underlying metabolic disturbance. Rapid correction of hyponatraemia can cause permanent neurological disability.

26. **D** ★★★

Approximately 50,000 children present to Emergency Departments with burns every year in the UK. Estimation of the area affected is an important part of the initial assessment, and is aided by the use of a Lund–Browder chart. Although fluid resuscitation in burns has been controversial, the Parkland formula is widely used in the management of paediatric burns. The take-home message is that fluid requirements are high because of losses through the damaged skin barrier.

Parkland formula

For the first 24 hours after the burn, give 4 mL/kg per % BSA burn of Hartmann's solution. Give half of this volume in the first 8 hours after the burn, and the other half in the next 16 hours.

27. E ★ ★ ★

There is no suggestion that there was significant intra-operative or post-operative bleeding, so major blood loss is unlikely. Iron-deficiency anaemia is a chronic pathology and would take longer than 24 hours to develop. Bone-marrow failure can result in anaemia, but is relatively rare and usually causes a pancytopenia, so it would be important to check the platelet and white cell counts, too. Most importantly, this patient has no features of profound anaemia, such as circulatory collapse (shock).

The most likely cause is a spurious result due to either an error when taking the blood sample (e.g. taking it from the drip arm and causing dilution) or a laboratory error (this is much less likely). As there are no features of circulatory compromise, a new sample should be taken and analysed.

→ www.surgical-tutor.org.uk/default-home.htm?core/preop1/anaemia.htm~right

28. E ★ ★ ★ ★   OHCS 9th edn → p. 777

The majority of organ donations in the UK occur from heart-beating donors. The use of non-heart-beating donors is increasing in the UK, but is still relatively uncommon. A patient does not have to be registered on the organ donor register to donate organs, but if they expressed the view that they would not want to donate organs during life, this decision is usually honoured. If a patient expressed the view that they wanted to donate their organs, but their living next of kin were against organ donation, it is unlikely that organs would be taken, as this would go against the relatives' wishes.

→ www.organdonation.nhs.uk

29. C ★ ★ ★ ★

Dexamethasone (a corticosteroid), 4–8 mg IV, is commonly used as an anti-emetic. It is usually given intra-operatively, as it is associated with unpleasant side-effects when given to patients who are awake.

30. B ★ ★ ★ ★

Anticholinergic drugs (e.g. hyoscine) are routinely used for their antisialagogue effect, particularly in the palliative care setting. Acetylcholine is the neurotransmitter at muscarinic receptors of the parasympathetic nervous system, responsible for control of secretions. Therefore anticholinergic drugs will block this pathway.

Extended Matching Questions

1. I ★

The combination of pinpoint pupils and shallow and infrequent respiration should alert you to opioid overdose.

2. D ★

Beta-blockers inhibit sympathetic effects on the heart and blood vessels, and cause severe bradycardia and hypotension in overdose.

3. K ★

This is the most common overdose that is seen acutely. Delayed presentation can cause potentially fatal liver damage, and the risk is worsened by concurrent alcohol consumption. Paracetamol hepatotoxicity is the commonest cause of acute liver failure in the UK.

4. F ★

Carbon monoxide toxicity can easily be missed, as patients appear pink and have oxygen saturations of 100% peripherally, due to the presence of carboxyhaemoglobin. Carbon monoxide has a significant affinity for haemoglobin, and also affects the release of oxygen to the tissues. In a patient with a suspicious history such as this, carboxyhaemoglobin levels must be measured.

5. G ★

Digoxin has a low therapeutic index and toxicity is common, especially in the elderly. Yellow vision (xanthopsia) is characteristic, together with nausea, anorexia, and confusion. Various ECG changes can occur.

6. B ★★★

Synchronized DC cardioversion is the treatment of choice for tachycardias with 'adverse signs' (e.g. chest pain, hypotension, or signs of heart failure).

→ www.resus.org.uk/pages/tachalgo.pdf

For patients who have not been successfully electrically cardioverted, anti-arrhythmic drugs are indicated. Amiodarone is widely used in this situation, but magnesium and lidocaine would also be first-line options. Correction of hypokalaemia and hypomagnesaemia is important, to allow the heart to restore sinus rhythm.

7. I ★★★

Anaphylaxis is managed by early administration of intramuscular epinephrine in the Emergency Department. In experienced hands (and with appropriate monitoring), epinephrine can be given intravenously and titrated to effect, but it can precipitate cardiac ischaemia and dangerous hypertension, which is why it is usually only given intravenously in cardiac arrest.

→ www.resus.org.uk/pages/reaction.pdf#search="anaphylaxis"

8. T ★★★

Although some of the other drugs listed here are indicated in asthma, setting up a nebulizer can be done quickly and easily and should be the first-line management.

9. D ★★★

The ECG signs indicate hyperkalaemia. The priority is to give a cardioprotective agent (calcium gluconate or calcium chloride).

10. C ★★★

This is the presentation of organophosphate poisoning, which classically presents with signs of a cholinergic syndrome. Organophosphate poisoning is a global problem which is seen more often in the developing world.

Organophosphates are phosphoric acid esters that are used in insecticides, herbicides, and also in nerve gas. They are highly toxic drugs that inhibit the enzyme acetylcholinesterase, which is responsible for the breakdown and recycling of acetylcholine. Consequently, the accumulation of the latter overstimulates the muscarinic receptors of the autonomic nervous system (i.e. parasympathetic system) and the nicotinic receptors of the skeletal muscles. This presents as excessive salivation, lacrimation, vomiting and diarrhoea, bradycardia, and bronchospasm, and is known as a cholinergic syndrome. In addition, the nicotinic stimulation causes muscle fasciculation followed by weakness, fatigue, and paralysis.

Management is supportive. Respiratory support may need to be provided if respiratory muscles are involved. Drug treatment includes atropine to antagonize acetylcholine at muscarinic receptors, and pralidoxime to reduce the extent of enzyme inhibition.

Chapter 9

Trauma and orthopaedics

Nev Davies

Over the years, trauma and orthopaedics has evolved into a vast specialty that is ever growing, with new technology, techniques, and implants. Computer-assisted surgery and minimally invasive approaches are current hot topics that are pushing the boundaries of delivering the best possible care for patients.

This specialty touches people of all ages from all walks of life. The practicality and logic in decision making and management appeal to today's modern 'orthopods.'

Trauma is a team specialty, and orthopaedic surgeons play an essential role in the initial and definitive management of patients with musculoskeletal injuries—saving life and saving limb.

Paediatric orthopaedics is a highly specialized area. However, as is the case for doctors in any setting, it is invaluable to have an understanding of the presentation of common paediatric orthopaedic conditions, such as developmental dysplasia of the hip and septic arthritis, which, if unrecognized can have serious consequences for the rest of the child's life.

Arthroplasty has been one of the true successes of the twenty-first century, and now over 140,000 knee and hip replacements are performed each year in the UK, revolutionizing the quality of life of patients with painful disabling arthritis.

To be a good orthopaedic surgeon requires not only a wide knowledge base, but also common sense, logic, and practical skills. *'A good surgeon knows how to operate; a great surgeon knows when to operate'* is a classic saying that was drilled into me as a young houseman. In this specialty there are often several management options facing the surgeon and the patient, and through careful discussion and the process of informed consent, a joint plan can be formulated and executed.

The questions in this chapter will help you to prepare both for your exams and for a future career as a doctor.

QUESTIONS

Single Best Answers

1. A 17-year-old man is knocked off his moped. He is wearing a helmet, and witnesses thought that he was travelling at 30 mph before impact. Which is the single most appropriate immediate management? ★

A Advanced Trauma Life Support (ATLS) assessment following guidelines

B CT scan of his head

C Glasgow Coma Scale assessment and pupil reaction

D Thorough mechanism of injury history and full examination

E X-rays of his chest, pelvis, and cervical spine

2. A motor cyclist has been involved in a motor vehicle collision. He is talking, has bruising on the right side of his chest but normal breath sounds, his pulse rate is 120 bpm, and his blood pressure is 60/40 mmHg. His Glasgow Coma Scale score is 15/15. He has bruising around his flanks and an obvious open fracture of his right tibia. He has blood at the urethral meatus. His chest X-ray shows some fractured ribs on the right, and his pelvic film is shown in Plate 9.1 (see Colour Plate section). Which is the single most appropriate next step in his management? ★

A Betadine-soaked dressing, IV antibiotics, and washout of his tibial fracture

B Chest drain for his rib fractures and potential haemothorax

C IV access, IV fluids, and blood replacement

D Pelvic external fixation

E Securing of a definitive airway with the anaesthetist

3. A 6-week-old baby with a 'clicky' hip is referred by the health visitor. She has had an ultrasound scan that confirms a dislocated right hip and a dysplastic acetabulum. Which single clinical finding best supports the diagnosis of a dislocated right hip? ★

A Asymmetrical skin creases on the thighs

B Clicking on abduction of the hip

C A dimple at the base of the spine

D Leg length discrepancy

E Limited abduction of the hip on the right

4. An 83-year-old man has had intermittent pain in the base of his spine for 4 months. It has become constant in nature and is not responding to simple analgesics. Which single factor in the history should alert you to the possibility of serious pathology? ★

A Night pain

B Past history of malignancy

C Sciatic pain radiating down the leg from the buttock to the foot

D Scoliosis

E Temperature of 38°C or more

5. A 30-year-old woman who is usually fit and well has had intermittent urinary incontinence and loss of sensation around her bottom for the last 24 hours. Which is the single most appropriate next step in management? ★

A Blood tests, spinal X-rays, and a urine dipstick

B History and examination, including a rectal examination

C Mobilization of the theatre team, as she needs to go straight to theatre

D Opiate analgesia and review by senior colleagues

E Urgent MRI scan of the spine

6. A 7-year-old boy has had an intermittent pain in his left hip for the past month. He walks with a slight limp and has decreased abduction at the hip joint. Which is the single most likely diagnosis? ★

A Juvenile idiopathic arthritis

B Missed developmental dysplasia of the hip

C Perthes' disease

D Slipped upper femoral epiphysis

E Transient synovitis

7. A 4-year-old boy has had pain and tenderness in his lower leg for 1 week. He is refusing to weight-bear. There is an area of swelling and warmth at the upper tibia, which is tender. He has a temperature of 39°C. His blood tests show:

- white cell count 30 × 10⁹/L
- erythrocyte sedimentation rate (ESR) 110 mm/hour
- C-reactive protein (CRP) 200 mg/L.

Which is the single most likely causative micro-organism? ★

A Kingella kingae

B Pseudomonas aeruginosa

C Salmonella paratyphi

D Staphylococcus aureus

E Staphylococcus epidermidis

8. A 70-year-old woman with rheumatoid arthritis is having a total knee replacement. Which is the single most important pre-operative investigation? ★

A Anteroposterior and lateral radiographs of the cervical spine

B Arterial blood gas analysis

C Dual-energy X-ray absorptiometry (DEXA) scanning

D Inflammatory markers

E Up-to-date anteroposterior and lateral X-rays of the knee

9. A 6-year-old boy is brought to the Emergency Department with a painful swollen arm. His mother is unsure what happened and gives a story of an unwitnessed fall off a bunk bed the day before. The boy has a lot of bruising all over his arm and upper body. Which is the single most appropriate management? ★

A Admit the child to the ward and contact your consultant

B Contact the duty social worker

C Discuss your concerns with the paediatrician on call

D Probe the mother about the cause of the bruises

E Send off a full blood count and clotting screen

10. A newborn baby has 'clicky' hips at birth. Which single feature is a risk factor for developmental dysplasia of the hip (DDH)? ★

A Family history of DDH

B Low birth weight

C Male gender

D Polyhydramnios

E Second sibling

11. A 45-year-old builder has pins and needles down the medial border of his forearm and weakness in the small muscles in his hand, causing him to drop things. Which is the single name and location of the nerve that is being compressed? ★

A Anterior interosseous nerve under the fibres of the flexor digitorum sublimis

B Median nerve in the carpal tunnel

C Posterior interosseous nerve under the proximal edge of the supinator muscle

D Ulnar nerve at the cubital tunnel

E Ulnar nerve in Guyon's canal

12. A 65-year-old man sustained a fracture of the femoral neck 4 years ago. He is undergoing a total hip replacement for collapse of the head and secondary osteoarthritis. He walks with a stick, and has an antalgic gait and a significant leg length discrepancy. Which is the single most likely benefit of the procedure? ★

A Equalization of the leg length discrepancy

B Improvement of walking distance

C Improvement of range of motion

D Pain relief

E Prevention of compensatory osteoarthritis in other joints

13. A 60-year-old man has a deformed painless right ankle and foot. He has had blistering and ulceration of his foot in the past. X-rays show a destructive Charcot-type arthropathy of the ankle and subtalar joints. Which is the single most likely underlying diagnosis? ★

A Alcohol-induced peripheral neuropathy

B Diabetes mellitus

C Hereditary motor and sensory neuropathy

D Leprosy

E Tertiary syphilis

14. A 9-year-old boy has put his arm through a glass door. There is significant bleeding from a 5 cm deep wound in his forearm. Which is the single most appropriate immediate management? ★

A Apply a high arm tourniquet

B Apply direct pressure over the axillary artery

C Apply direct pressure over the wound

D Give IV antibiotics and tetanus prophylaxis

E Give local anaesthetic and clip the bleeding vessel

15. A 25-year-old man has been involved in a drunken brawl and has been stabbed in the chest. He is tachypnoeic, tachycardic, and hypotensive, and has two wounds in the left thorax. Which is the single most appropriate immediate management? ★

A Apply direct pressure over the stab wounds to stem the bleeding

B Fast bleep the cardiothoracic surgeons

C Obtain IV access and cross-match 6 units of blood

D Open the airway and give high-flow oxygen

E Open the chest (thoracotomy) and begin internal cardiac massage

16. A 7-year-old boy has an open fracture of his forearm. He is on a scout trip away from home and attends the hospital with his scout leader. You need to take him to theatre immediately, but are unable to contact his parents, who are away on holiday. Which is the single most appropriate course of action? ★

A Ask a duty social worker to sign the consent form

B Ask another doctor to sign the consent form

C Ask the boy to sign the consent form

D Ask the scout leader to sign the consent form

E Written consent is not required as this is an emergency

17. A 75-year-old man attends his 6-week follow-up appointment after a primary right total hip replacement for osteoarthritis. He walks in with the aid of one stick and, as he walks, his upper body sways to the right when he stands on his operated leg. Which is the single best description of his altered gait? ★

A Antalgic

B Normal for this stage in his post-operative recovery

C Short leg

D Trendelenburg positive

E Varus thrust

18. A 36-year-old computer programmer has a painful lump on the volar aspect of his wrist. The lump is well defined, fluctuant, and pulsatile, but it does not transilluminate. Which is the single most appropriate next step in management? ★

A Aspirate the lump in the clinic under local anaesthetic, and inject steroid

B Explain the benign nature of the lump and that it is likely to resolve spontaneously with time

C Organize an ultrasound scan to confirm the diagnosis

D Put the patient on the waiting list for excision of the lump under general anaesthetic

E Put the patient on the waiting list for excision of the lump under local anaesthetic

19. A 60-year-old woman has sustained a low-energy fracture of the distal radius. Last year she fell and sustained a proximal femoral fracture, which was fixed with a dynamic hip screw. A recent DEXA scan has shown a T score of −3. Which is the single most likely diagnosis? ★ ★

A Oligodystrophy

B Osteomalacia

C Osteopenia

D Osteopetrosis

E Osteoporosis

20. A patient is concerned about the risk of deep infection following primary total hip replacement. Which single factor has had the greatest impact on reducing joint replacement infection? ★ ★

A Antibiotic-loaded cement

B Body-exhaust suits for the surgeons

C Disposable gowns

D Laminar air flow systems

E Peri-operative prophylactic systemic antibiotics

21. A 60-year-old woman has had neck pain for several years. She now has an acute prolapse of the C5/6 disc, causing nerve root compression on the right side. Which single set of symptoms and signs is she most likely to have? ★ ★

A Dysaesthesia in the thumb and index finger, and weakness of elbow extension

B Increased tone and hyper-reflexia in the right arm

C None of these

D Pain and numbness in the medial forearm

E Weakness of elbow flexion and loss of triceps reflex

22. A 2-year-old girl has had multiple bony fractures since birth. She has discoloured teeth, poor growth, and blue sclera. Which is the single most likely diagnosis? ★ ★

A Achondroplasia

B Craniocleidodysostosis

C Hypophosphatasia

D Osteogenesis imperfecta

E Osteopetrosis

23. A 50-year-old man has increasing pain in his right knee. The pain is not controlled by daily ibuprofen and paracetamol, and he is particularly troubled by it when going up and down stairs. He experiences pain even when at rest. He had a total meniscectomy 30 years ago after a football injury when he also ruptured his anterior cruciate ligament. His X-ray is shown in Plate 9.2 (see Colour Plate section). Which is the single most appropriate management? ★ ★

A Increase his pain medications and advise him to use a stick

B Medial unicompartmental knee replacement

C Referral for physiotherapy

D Steroid injection and review

E Total knee replacement

24. A 25-year-old man has been knocked off his motorcycle. He has an open fracture of his femur. His leg X-ray is shown in Plate 9.3 (see Colour Plate section). Which is the single most appropriate definitive management? ★ ★

A External fixator with washout and debridement of the wound and delayed primary closure

B Intramedullary nail with washout and debridement of the wound and delayed primary closure

C Open reduction and plate fixation with washout and debridement of the wound and primary closure

D Washout and debridement of the wound and application of a Thomas splint

E Washout and debridement of the wound and a long leg cast with a window for a vacuum suction pump

25. A baby has been born with a foot deformity, as shown in Plate 9.4 (see Colour Plate section). Which is the single best description of this foot deformity? ★ ★

A Calcaneous, abductus, valgus

B Cavus, adductus, varus, equinus

C Cavus, calcaneous, adductus, varus

D Cavus, valgus, equinus

E Pes planus

26. A 26-year-old man who plays squash socially presents with a 4-month history of unilateral heel pain. He has circumferential thickening of the Achilles tendon 2 cm proximal to its insertion at the os calcis, and is unable to perform a tiptoe test. Which is the single most likely diagnosis? ★ ★

A Achilles insertional tendonitis

B Chronic Achilles tendon rupture

C Hagland's deformity of the os calcis

D Retrocalcaneal bursitis

E Tibialis posterior tendonitis

27. A 79-year-old woman has fallen at home. She has hip pain and a short and externally rotated left leg. Radiographs show a displaced intracapsular fracture of her left neck of femur. Previously she walked outdoors independently with the aid of a stick. She is otherwise medically fit. Which is the single most appropriate surgical management? ★ ★

A Cemented hemiarthroplasty

B Dynamic hip screw and plate

C Total hip replacement

D Uncemented hemiarthroplasty

E Three divergent cannulated screws

28. A 20-year-old man falls off his motorbike and fractures his tibial shaft. The management options are discussed with him and he opts for an intramedullary nail. He is put into a backslab cast and listed for surgery the next day. His leg is kept strictly elevated. At 3.30 am he develops increasing pain despite morphine treatment. Which is the single most appropriate next step in management? ★ ★ ★

A Add a non-steroidal anti-inflammatory drug to his pain relief, and review in 30 minutes

B Call the anaesthetist to set up a patient-controlled morphine analgesia system

C Call your senior colleague, as the patient needs to go to theatre immediately

D List the patient for theatre at 6 am, when his stomach will be empty and it will be safe to give him an anaesthetic

E Split his cast to skin, continue elevation, and review him with a senior colleague in 15 minutes

29. A 93-year-old woman is bed-bound in a nursing home and has severe dementia. She has fallen out of bed. Her right hip is stiff but painless, and an X-ray reveals a dislocated total hip replacement (THR). She also has a large 10 × 5 cm open pre-tibial laceration. She has a respiratory rate of 23 breaths/minute, with evidence of ischaemic changes on the ECG. Which is the single most appropriate specialty to call for help with the management of this patient? ★ ★ ★

A Anaesthetist, to give a general anaesthetic to reduce the THR

B Cardiologist, to help to interpret the ECG changes

C General medical team, to optimize medical care prior to any intervention

D Plastic surgeon, to help to manage the open pre-tibial laceration

E Psychiatrist, to assess whether the patient can consent to treatment

30. A 35-year-old man was playing five-a-side football when he thought he had been kicked in the back of the leg. The next day he is hobbling and has pain and swelling around his Achilles tendon. Simmonds' test is equivocal. Which is the single most appropriate investigation to confirm the diagnosis and plan further management? ★ ★ ★ ★

A CT scan

B Examination under anaesthetic

C MRI scan

D Plain X-ray

E Ultrasound scan

31. A 25-year-old man with epilepsy has a painful swollen shoulder after having a fit earlier that day. X-rays are taken, as shown in Plate 9.5 (see Colour Plate section). Which is the single most appropriate management? ★ ★ ★ ★

A Arrange for a CT scan to help to plan operative management

B Arrange for the patient to go to theatre for a closed reduction

C Arrange for the patient to go to theatre for an open reduction

D Perform reduction using the Hippocratic method under sedation

E Perform reduction using Kocher's method under sedation

32. A 45-year-old woman has an oblique fracture of her distal fibula. Which is the single best technique to compress the two fragments of bone? ★ ★ ★ ★

A Dynamic compression plate and cancellous screws

B Elastic titanium intramedullary nails

C External fixation with supplementary K-wire fixation

D Lag screw and neutralization plate

E Locking plate with locking screws

33. A 60-year-old man has an acutely painful swollen knee. In total, 100 mL of synovial fluid are aspirated. The fluid is straw-coloured and viscous. Analysis shows no crystals, and a white cell count of $4000/mm^3$ with neutrophils < 25%. The patient reports that his pain is much improved after aspiration. Which is the single most likely diagnosis? ★ ★ ★ ★

A Gout

B Pseudogout

C Reactive arthritis

D Rheumatoid arthritis

E Septic arthritis

34. A 45-year-old man has fallen 20 feet off a ladder. As he fell, his right leg became caught in the rungs of the ladder and he felt his knee 'pop in and pop out.' He has a very swollen tender knee with a cool white limb and a very faint dorsalis pedis pulse. Which is the single most appropriate immediate management? ★ ★ ★ ★

A Anteroposterior and lateral lower limb radiographs

B Mobilize the theatre team immediately, as the patient needs to undergo an open exploration of the popliteal vessels

C MRI of the patient's knee to determine which ligaments are damaged

D Organize an arteriogram and contact the vascular surgeons for an urgent review

E Organize an urgent fasciotomy to prevent compartment syndrome

35. A 65-year-old man has undergone a primary total hip replacement for osteoarthritis. Post-operatively, he has developed a foot drop, with numbness in his foot and weakness of ankle dorsiflexion to 2/5 power. Which is the single most likely cause of the foot drop? ★ ★ ★ ★

A Axonotmesis of the common peroneal nerve at the head of the fibula due to pressure from positioning during the procedure

B Axonotmesis of the sciatic nerve due to intra-operative traction injury secondary to misplaced retractors

C Neuropraxia of the common peroneal nerve at the head of the fibula due to pressure from positioning during the procedure

D Neuropraxia of the sciatic nerve due to intra-operative traction injury secondary to misplaced retractors

E Neuronotmesis of the sciatic nerve during surgery

36. A 15-year-old boy has fractured his humerus. His X-ray is shown in Plate 9.6 (see Colour Plate section). Which is the single most likely mechanism of injury? ★ ★ ★ ★

A Bending force

B Bending force with axial compression

C Direct impact from lateral aspect

D Direct impact from medial aspect

E Torsional force

37. A 13-year-old boy has had repeated ankle sprains, midfoot pain, and problems walking on uneven ground. He has a flat foot that does not correct into varus when he stands on tiptoe. He also has a stiff subtalar joint. Which is the single most likely diagnosis? ★ ★ ★ ★

A Charcot–Marie–Tooth disease

B Lateral ligament insufficiency (ankle)

C Physiological flexible flat foot

D Sever's disease

E Tarsal coalition

38. A 50-year-old diabetic man has recurrent triggering of the ring finger. The finger is stuck in flexion. It was injected 2 years ago with good results. Which is the single most appropriate management? ★ ★ ★ ★

A Operative release under general anaesthetic

B Operative release under local anaesthetic

C Repeat of the injection

D Stretching and a night splint with physiotherapy

E Ultrasound scan to confirm the diagnosis

39. A 22-year-old footballer ruptures his anterior cruciate ligament and tears his medial meniscus after twisting his knee in training. Which single group of clinical findings is most likely 2 weeks after the initial injury? ★ ★ ★ ★

A Effusion, hyperextension, and generalized joint-line tenderness

B Effusion, medial joint-line tenderness, and positive Lachman's test

C Increased opening on valgus stress, and tenderness medially

D Increased posterior sag, positive anterior draw, and negative Lachman's test

E Quadriceps wasting, extensor lag, and positive Lachman's test

Extended Matching Questions

Nerve supply of the arm

For each anatomical description, choose the *single* most likely nerve from the list of options below. Each option may be used once, more than once, or not at all. ★

A Anterior interosseous nerve

B Axillary nerve

C Medial cutaneous nerve of forearm

D Median nerve

E Musculocutaneous nerve

F Posterior interosseus nerve

G Radial nerve

H Superficial radial nerve

I Ulnar nerve

1. It is found medial to the coracoid process and in close relationship to the conjoint tendon. It supplies the biceps brachii and muscles of the anterior compartment of the upper arm.

2. It is the motor supply of the extensor compartment of the forearm and wrist.

3. It is at risk from injury on the medial border of the elbow. It supplies the small muscles of the hand.

4. It is found in close relationship to the humeral head. It can be injured by glenohumeral joint dislocation.

5. It lies in close relationship to the humeral diaphysis in the spiral groove. It is at risk in humeral shaft fractures.

Causes of bone tumours

For each patient with a bony tumour, choose the *single* most likely diagnosis from the list of options below. Each option may be used once, more than once, or not at all. ★ ★

A Aneurysmal bone cyst

B Chondrosarcoma

C Chordoma

D Ewing's sarcoma

E Giant-cell tumour

F Metastatic lesion

G Osteochondroma

H Osteoid osteoma

I Osteosarcoma

J Soft tissue sarcoma

6. An 80-year-old man has had Paget's disease for 10 years. He now has increasing pain and swelling in his distal femur.

7. A 15-year-old boy has severe night pain in his upper thigh, which responds well to aspirin.

8. A 17-year-old woman has pain and local warmth in her lower thigh. An X-ray shows an expansile lytic lesion, and an MRI scan shows that it contains multiple fluid-filled levels.

9. An 80-year-old woman with renal-cell carcinoma has a hard fixed breast lump and excruciating lower back pain.

10. A 65-year-old man has had lower back pain, impotence, and tenesmus for several months. He now has acute urinary retention.

Causes of shoulder problems

For each patient with a shoulder problem, choose the *single* most likely diagnosis from the list of options below. Each option may be used once, more than once, or not at all. ★ ★

A Acromioclavicular joint osteoarthritis

B Calcific tendonitis

C Frozen shoulder

D Glenohumeral joint osteoarthritis

E Impingement

F Long head of biceps tendon rupture

G Painful arc syndrome

H Rotator cuff full-thickness tear

I Supraspinatus tendonitis

11. A 30-year-old woman has an acute onset of continuous pain in the shoulder, radiating down the arm. It is so severe that she requires opiate analgesia.

12. An 80-year-old man has global decreased range of motion of the shoulder and night pain.

13. A 65-year-old man has good power in his shoulders but an asymmetrical appearance of the musculature of his upper arms.

14. A 45-year-old woman has a vague story of a bang on the arm. She now has stiffness and inability to sleep on her bad side.

15. A 75-year-old retired farmer has weakness in forward elevation and abduction of his shoulder, although it can be moved passively through the complete range.

Causes of hand and wrist problems

For each patient with pain in the hand, choose the *single* most likely diagnosis from the list of options below. Each option may be used once, more than once, or not at all. ★ ★ ★ ★

A Atypical carpal tunnel syndrome

B Carpometacarpal osteoarthritis

C De Quervain's tenosynovitis

D Distal radial fracture

E Flexor carpi radialis tendonitis

F Ganglion

G Intersection syndrome

H Scaphoid fracture

I Scaphotrapeziotrapezoid osteoarthritis

J Ulnar collateral ligament injury of the thumb

16. A 35-year-old man falls at the dry ski slope on to an outstretched hand. His thumb is swollen and painful to move, and there is minimal tenderness at the base of the thumb.

17. A 55-year-old woman has pain at the base of both thumbs. Radiographs show loss of joint space and sclerosis at the joint between the first metacarpal and the trapezium.

18. A 40-year-old woman has tenderness and a soft fullness at the base of the anatomical snuffbox of the thumb. There is no history of trauma.

19. A 65-year-old woman falls on to her dominant hand. She has bruising and global tenderness all around the wrist.

20. A 55-year-old woman has had pain at the base of the thumb for a week. Extension against resistance exacerbates the pain, as does palpation over the first dorsal extensor compartment.

Causes of hip and knee problems in children

For each child with pain, choose the *single* most likely diagnosis from the list of options below. Each option may be used once, more than once, or not at all. ★ ★ ★ ★

A Developmental dysplasia of the hip

B Ewing's sarcoma of the pelvis

C Idiopathic coxa vara

D Juvenile idiopathic arthritis

E Perthes' disease

F Septic arthritis

G Slipped upper femoral epiphysis

H Transient synovitis

21. A 7-year-old boy has intermittent pain in his right hip. He is well in himself but has a reduced range of movement, with irritability at the extremes of motion.

22. A 3-year-old girl has a limp. She has a leg length discrepancy of 2 cm, shorter on the left, asymmetrical skin creases, and marked limitation in abduction of the left hip.

23. A 13-year-old boy has pain in the groin. It was intermittent at first, but is becoming more constant and wakes him up at night. He had a retinoblastoma as a baby.

24. A 6-year-old boy has had intermittent pain, stiffness, and swelling of the knee over the last year. There is an effusion and limitation of flexion.

25. A 12-year-old boy who weighs 75 kg has a painful knee and a limp.

ANSWERS

Single Best Answers

1. A ★   OHCS 9th edn → p. 724

Advanced Trauma Life Support (ATLS) guidelines are regarded as the international gold standard for the initial management of the traumatized patient.

→ www.rcseng.ac.uk/education/courses/atls.html/?searchterm=ATLS

2. C ★

In keeping with any significant injury, the immediate priority is to ensure that airway, breathing, and circulation are not compromised. This man's airway and breathing seem to be secure, so you should go on to treat the potential blood loss from the pelvic fracture by securing circulation.

3. E ★   OHCS 9th edn → pp. 684–685

Clicking and asymmetry of skin creases are 'soft' signs of hip dislocation. The limitation of abduction suggests a positive Ortolani's test, which means that the hip is out of joint posteriorly.

4. B ★   OHCS 9th edn → p. 678

This suggests that spinal metastases may be the cause. The other features may also be present with metastatic lesions, but can be features of other diagnoses. Night pain can indicate significant pathology and should be taken seriously.

5. B ★   OHCS 9th edn → p. 675

This history suggests cauda equina syndrome, of which there are many causes. However, the young age makes a sinister cause unlikely. The first step is always a thorough history and examination, and a rectal examination must always be performed to assess anal tone.

6. C ★   OHCS 9th edn → p. 682

In this age group, the most important cause of persistent limp is Perthes' disease, which is an avascular necrosis of the femoral head. Slipped upper femoral epiphysis tends to occur in older overweight children. Transient synovitis should not last for a month. Dysplasia of the hip would have been seen at an earlier age than 7 years. Juvenile idiopathic arthritis is possible but less likely.

7. D ★   OHCS 9th edn → p. 696

This is a picture of osteomyelitis, commonly caused by *Staphylococcus aureus*.

8. A ★   OHCS 9th edn → pp. 613–614

Guidelines exist that recommend which pre-operative investigations should be performed. However, patients with rheumatoid arthritis are at risk of cervical involvement, which can make anaesthetic management of the neck and airway difficult. If in doubt, always discuss the case with an anaesthetist.

→ www.nice.org.uk/nicemedia/pdf/CG3NICEguideline.pdf

9. C ★   OHCS 9th edn → p. 146

Any doctor who sees children needs to be aware of the possibility of non-accidental injury. However, although it is important to document exactly what you have found, specialist paediatric doctors should be involved in these cases. They can work with the parent specialty team to gather further information and plan appropriate management.

10. A ★   OHCS 9th edn → p. 684

The risk factors for DDH are as follows:

• Female gender
• Firstborn
• Foot first (breech)
• Family history
• Further bony abnormalities (e.g. talipes equinovarus).

11. D ★   OHCS 9th edn → p. 668

12. D ★   OHCS 9th edn → p. 706

The main benefit of hip replacement is pain control. It is much less successful in improving mobility.

13. B ★

This patient's age makes hereditary motor and sensory neuropathy unlikely. Diabetes is the commonest cause of neuropathy, leading to arthropathy.

14. C ★

Following ABC (airway, breathing, and circulation) guidelines, the first step in controlling bleeding is the application of direct pressure. Once the bleeding is under control, this patient may need further surgical intervention, and antibiotics and tetanus prophylaxis may be indicated, but these are not the priorities.

15. D ★

Following Advanced Trauma Life Support (ATLS) guidelines, securing an airway is always the first priority.

16. E ★

Only a person with parental responsibility can give valid consent on behalf of a child who is not Gillick competent. In some cases the parent may sign over parental responsibility to another adult, but usually this does not happen. In an emergency, the doctor should document the need for an emergency procedure clearly, and state why it is needed, but can proceed to save life or limb without formal written consent.

17. D ★   OHCS 9th edn → p. 680

The Trendelenburg test assesses the stability of the hip. When the patient stands on the affected leg, the pelvis falls on the opposite side, causing the upper body to lurch to the affected side in order to compensate. This is a positive test. It is caused by weak abductor muscles, a dislocated hip, or the absence of a stable fulcrum.

18. C ★   OHCS 9th edn → p. 668

This is the classic location and description of a ganglion—that is, a benign bulge of synovium. It may resolve spontaneously, but if it is painful, it can be aspirated or excised. However, diagnosis should be confirmed first with soft-tissue imaging.

19. E ★ ★

DEXA stands for dual-energy X-ray absorptiometry, and is considered to be the most accurate test for bone density. Although standard X-rays show changes in bone density after about 40% bone loss, a DEXA scan can detect changes after about a 1% change. The results of a DEXA scan are reported in two ways—as T scores and as Z scores. A T score compares bone density with the optimal peak bone density for gender. It is reported as the number of standard deviations below the mean. A T score of greater than –1 is considered to be normal. A T score of –1 to –2.5 is considered to be osteopenia and the patient is at risk of developing osteoporosis. A T score of less than –2.5 is diagnostic of osteoporosis.

20. **E** ★ ★

21. **A** ★ ★   OHCS 9th edn → pp. 660, 716–7, 762–3

Knowledge of the specific patterns of nerve damage is useful in diagnosis (see the tables and pictures in OHCS 9th edn).

22. **D** ★ ★

These are the features of some types of osteogenesis imperfecta, a rare cause of multiple fractures. These signs may help to raise suspicion of the diagnosis.

23. **E** ★ ★   OHCS 9th edn → p. 706

For this patient, non-operative measures for management of his osteo-arthritis have been exhausted, and surgical treatment is warranted. His X-ray shows medial compartment osteoarthritis. However, he requires a total knee replacement because a unicompartmental knee replacement is contraindicated in a patient without an anterior cruciate ligament.

24. **B** ★ ★   OHCS 9th edn → p. 752

Intramedullary nails align and stabilize the bone and share the load with the bone. They allow early mobilization. Because the fracture is open, it requires careful washing out. Delayed primary closure refers to the initial debridement and then closing of the wound at a later stage. This allows better healing of contaminated wounds.

25. **B** ★ ★   OHCS 9th edn → p. 684

This is an image of club foot, or talipes equinovarus. A full club foot involves the ankle (talus) and foot (pes), and is equinus (the heel is ele-vated like that of a horse) and cavus (with an exaggerated arch). It is varus (turned inward) and adducted (moved towards the midline). It cannot be moved through the normal range of movements, and the Achilles tendon is tight and the calf muscle shortened.

26. B ★ ★

This question requires you to correctly identify the Achilles tendon as the source of the pathology. Patients with tibialis posterior tendonitis also find it difficult to stand on tiptoe. Circumferential thickening could be due to chronic rupture or tendonitis. Retrocalcaneal bursitis tenderness tends to be located more distally, behind the tendon.

27. C ★★

Intracapsular fractures require either a total hip replacement or hemi-arthroplasty. Patients who were able to walk independently outside with the aid of no more than a stick, who are not cognitively impaired, and who are medically fit for anaesthesia and surgery should be offered a total hip replacement.

National Institute for Health and Clinical Excellence (2011). *Hip Fracture: the management of hip fracture in adults.* NICE Clinical Guideline, CG124:

→ http://guidance.nice.org.uk/CG124

28. E ★★★   OHCS 9th edn → p. 734

Patients with leg fractures are at risk of developing compartment syndrome, inflammation, and swelling within a closed fascial compartment, leading to impaired blood supply. However, this man is in a cast, so simple relief of the external pressure and elevation may alleviate the pain and swelling. If the pain continues, he may be developing compartment syndrome and require fasciotomy, so a close review is essential.

29. C ★★★

This situation is not uncommon. The patient is more likely to suffer harm as a result of her medical illness than in relation to her dislocated THR, and medical problems should be co-managed with medical teams in the interest of best outcome for the patient.

30. E ★★★★   OHCS 9th edn → p. 712

A ruptured Achilles tendon causes sudden pain when running or jumping, and the heel cannot be raised from the floor when the patient is standing on the affected leg. In Simmonds' test, the patient kneels on a chair and the calf is squeezed; there will be less plantar flexion of the foot on the affected side. An ultrasound scan is the easiest and most discriminatory test for soft-tissue injuries, although it is operator dependent.

31. A ★★★★   OHCS 9th edn → p. 740

The radiographs show a locked posterior dislocation of the glenohumeral joint. This injury is often missed, as the signs (positive 'light-bulb' sign) are subtle on the anteroposterior view. The diagnosis is obvious on the axillary view. This is a difficult problem, and often further imaging is necessary to plan surgical management.

32. D ★★★★   OHCS 9th edn → p. 754

A lag screw is the best technique for producing interfragmentary compression in the context of absolute stability. This allows the fracture to heal by primary bone healing without the formation of a callus.

33. C ★★★★ OHCS 9th edn → pp. 708–709

Analysis of the colour, viscosity, and composition of synovial fluid is important. In this patient the straw colour and high viscosity but low number of neutrophils point to a non-inflammatory cause. In patients with inflammation or infection, the fluid is yellow with a high number of neutrophils.

34. D ★★★★

The history and examination findings should alert you to a possible knee dislocation that has self-reduced. This poses a significant risk to the neurovascular bundle. An arteriogram is the gold-standard investigation, with an urgent review by the vascular surgeons.

35. D ★★★★

Neuropraxia (physiological conduction block) is the most common type of nerve injury encountered, usually due to compression on the nerve. In total hip replacement, misplaced retractors are the usual cause of this, and the sciatic nerve is the most commonly involved nerve. Neuropraxia is often explained to patients as 'bruising to the nerve.' Nerve function usually returns to normal, although this can take many months.

36. E ★★★★

This is a spiral fracture, which is caused by a twisting force.

37. E ★★★★

Tarsal coalition—an abnormal connection between the tarsal bones—commonly presents in adolescence as the connection ossifies with growth of the child. Often there is a history of repeated ankle sprains and difficulty walking on uneven ground.

38. B ★★★★ OHCS 9th edn → p. 668

Diabetics are renowned for having recurrent resistant triggering digits. Operative release under local anaesthetic avoids the complications of a general anaesthetic (which are increased in a diabetic patient), and allows the surgeon to check the release by asking the patient to move the finger intra-operatively.

39. B ★★★★ OHCS 9th edn → p. 686

This patient is likely to have a residual effusion 2 weeks after a significant knee injury. Joint-line tenderness is a non-specific examination finding in a knee with intra-articular damage. Lachman's test, performed with the knee in 30° of flexion, is the most sensitive clinical test for diagnosing an anterior cruciate ligament injury. Important points are to compare with the other knee and the presence or absence of an end point.

Extended Matching Questions

1. **E** ★

2. **F** ★

3. **I** ★

4. **B** ★

5. **G** ★

General feedback on 1–5: OHCS 9th edn → p. 762
→ www.instantanatomy.net/arm/nerves/general.html
→ www.surgical-tutor.org.uk/default-home.htm

---

6. **I** ★★

7. **H** ★★

8. **A** ★★

9. **F** ★★

10. **C** ★★

General feedback on 6–10: OHCS 9th edn → pp. 698–699
Bone tumours can be benign or malignant. Most malignant bone tumours are metastases from distant primaries. Even benign bone tumours can cause pain, swelling, and fractures.

Osteosarcoma is the commonest primary bone malignancy, and typically occurs in growing areas of bone. Although it is most frequently found in teenagers, Paget's disease, the increased production of new bone, is a risk factor. In this case, the pain and swelling would increase. Ewing's sarcoma is also a primary malignant tumour that typically occurs in the pelvis and long bones in teenagers. Chondrosarcomas arise from cartilage, occur in the axial skeleton of middle-aged people, and present with a lump. Giant-cell tumour is an osteolytic lesion that again typically occurs around the epiphyses of young adults. Metastases tend to occur in the spine, ribs, and pelvis. Breast, prostate, lung, kidney, and colon carcinomas all spread to bone. Chordoma is a rare slow-growing bone malignancy that develops in remnants of the embryonic notochord. It typically occurs at the base of the spine or skull and causes compression of the spinal cord.

Benign tumours include osteochondroma, which is a cartilaginous overgrowth that causes a painless lump. Osteoid osteoma presents as a painful area, often in the tibia or femur, and often causes night pain that is relieved by non-steroidal anti-inflammatory drugs.

An aneurysmal bone cyst is an expansile osteolytic lesion that may arise in tumours or following a bone injury. It can arise in any bone, and typically causes fairly rapid development of pain and local swelling, with local skin warmth and restricted joint movement. It appears cystic on imaging.

11. B ★★

This is a build-up of calcium in the rotator cuff tendons, which is acutely painful and probably one of the most painful conditions that can occur in the shoulder. It can also cause impingement when lifting the arm.

12. D ★★

Osteoarthritis in the shoulder is less common than in other joints, but the risk increases with age and previous injury. The pain and stiffness are progressive and limit movement in all directions.

13. F ★★

This feels like 'something going' when it happens, and causes a golf-ball-like swelling in the biceps on flexion of the elbow.

14. C ★★

A 'frozen shoulder' refers to a condition in which the shoulder is almost completely immovable due to inflammation of the capsule and ligaments. It may be triggered by injury. There is a phase of pain and progressive loss of motion, followed by resolution of the pain with worsening stiffness that may take a couple of years to resolve.

15. H ★★

Specific limitation of movement leads to the relevant anatomy. Shoulder movement is complex and is controlled by several muscles, which come into play at different points in movement. Tears in tendons in the rotator cuff limit active movement.

General feedback on 11–15: OHCS 9th edn → pp. 662–664
→ www.shoulderdoc.co.uk

16. J ★★★★

The ulnar collateral ligament is typically injured by a fall on to a hand with the thumb spread out, causing it to bend back. It causes pain and swelling at the base of the thumb, where the metacarpophalangeal joint is located. This condition is also known as 'gamekeeper's thumb'.

17. B ★★★★

Osteoarthritis is common, and typical findings are loss of joint space and sclerosis on X-ray.

18. F ★★★★

A ganglion is a soft-tissue benign swelling that occurs on or around the joints or tendons in the hand and foot.

19. D ★★★★

A fall on to an outstretched hand can cause damage anywhere along the arm from the thumb to the shoulder, depending on factors such as age and the mechanism of injury. The location of swelling, pain, and bruising indicates the area of damage. In post-menopausal women, wrist fractures are common after falls.

20. C ★★★★

This is inflammation of the tendons at the base of the thumb. It causes localized pain and swelling. Finkelstein's manoeuvre is worsening of pain when the thumb is folded across the palm and the fingers are folded over the top.

General feedback on 16–20: OHCS 9th edn → pp. 742–746

21. E ★★★★

This osteochondritis of the femoral head presents in children aged 3–11 years, and in boys more often than in girls. It causes limitation of movement in all directions.

22. A ★★★★

Despite neonatal screening, dislocated hips are still missed. As in this case, children may walk late or with a limp.

23. B ★★★★

Pain that wakes a person at night should always be taken seriously. In this case, the past history of a malignancy should raise concern about another malignancy. Ewing's sarcoma usually presents in adolescence.

24. D ★ ★ ★ ★

The story of recurrent pain and swelling suggests a chronic condition. Juvenile idiopathic arthritis is an inflammatory arthritis, so will cause effusion, warmth, and limited movement.

25. G ★ ★ ★ ★

This occurs in peripubertal overweight children, and in boys more often than in girls. It causes limping and pain in the groin or knee, although these may be mild.

General feedback on 20–25: OHCS 9th edn → pp. 682, 684, 698

Chapter 10

Emergency medicine

Ruth Brown

Emergency medicine is not all 'ER', glamour, and fast-moving action. Much of it requires caring for relatively minor problems or complex elderly patients. A solid knowledge of basic sciences is essential to support the clinical and practical management decisions, and you need to know the acute presentations of all specialties. This requires a great deal of study as well as a sensible approach to finding information on unknown conditions while you are working. No one can know everything, but having a system for approaching a problem and applying basic principles helps.

Gathering information rapidly is important. Gaining clues from the patient and their relative(s) is useful, as is obtaining information on events at the scene from the ambulance paramedics. Hospital notes are often not available and neither is the GP, so you have to make decisions on the basis of limited information. Rather than making definitive diagnoses confirmed by expensive tests, the role of the emergency physician is to determine the immediate threat to life or limb and to treat that threat, while gathering information to make a 'most likely' diagnosis so that treatment can be started. Observing the patient in a clinical decision unit can often help to confirm your suspicions, give you further information on how severe a condition is, or eliminate a possible diagnosis.

Ultimately, emergency medicine requires the assessment of risk, evaluation of the added benefit of admission over discharge, and excellent communication. The only way to learn emergency medicine is to practise, to discuss patients, and to develop your analytical and decision-making skills. The following questions are designed to develop some of these skills, by showing you an approach to solving the clinical problems that are commonly encountered in the Emergency Department, how to use tests efficiently and effectively, and some of the options for treatment that are available other than admission under inpatient teams.

QUESTIONS

Single Best Answers

1. A 24-year-old man is hit by a car travelling at 50 mph. He is unconscious at the scene and there are only two rescuers. He has an obvious fracture of his right leg and swelling of his abdomen. Which is the single most appropriate immediate management of this patient's assumed cervical spine injury at the scene? ★

A Collar, sandbags, and tape

B Halo traction

C Manual in-line immobilization

D Manual in-line traction

E Soft sponge collar

2. A 46-year-old woman is in a coma. Her partner tells you that she has had abdominal pain and vomiting for 3 days. She is clinically dehydrated. Her blood sugar level is 48 mmol/L and her arterial pH is 7.0. Which is the single most appropriate immediate management? ★

A Bolus of normal saline

B IV cefuroxime and metronidazole

C Infusion of short-acting insulin at 10 U/hour

D Normal saline 2 L with potassium 40 mmol/L over 4 hours

E IV prochlorperazine

3. A 45-year-old man has a 2 cm laceration to the radial border of the middle and distal phalanx of his right index finger. Which is the single most appropriate local anaesthetic to use to close the wound? ★

A 0.5% bupivacaine without epinephrine (adrenaline)

B 1% lidocaine with epinephrine (adrenaline) 1:1000

C 1% lidocaine without epinephrine (adrenaline)

D 2% lidocaine with epinephrine (adrenaline) 1:1000

E 5% prilocaine without epinephrine (adrenaline)

4. A 40-year-old woman has pain and discharge from her right ear, a temperature of 38.3°C, a blocked nose, and a mild cough. She had a slight pain and deafness in her right ear 1 week ago, which she treated with warm olive oil dripped into her ear. She is a telebanking operator who uses a headset with an earpiece in her right ear. Which is the single most likely diagnosis? ★

A Extensive wax in the ear

B Foreign body in the ear

C Otitis externa

D Otitis media

E Perforated eardrum

5. A 56-year-old man has had a fall. He has a fracture of the radial head, which is undisplaced. Which is the single most appropriate method of immobilizing this fracture? ★

A Above-arm back slab

B Broad arm sling

C Collar and cuff

D Futura splint

E High arm sling

6. An 85-year-old man has an epistaxis. He is on warfarin for atrial fibrillation. Which single drug that he has recently been started on is most likely to be related to the cause of the epistaxis? ★

A Aspirin

B Bendroflumethiazide

C Clopidogrel

D Erythromycin

E Penicillin

7. An 89-year-old woman has had multiple falls. She has been to the Emergency Department 30 times in the last 6 months, but has only been admitted once. You assess her and can find little acutely wrong with her, but are concerned about sending her home. She appears to be unsteady on her feet. Which single service would be most helpful in contributing to a management plan? ★

A GP

B Hospital chiropody

C Hospital optician

D Medical registrar

E Occupational therapy

8. A 72-year-old man is brought to the Emergency Department in shock. His systolic blood pressure is 76 mmHg, with a pulse rate of 120 bpm. He has a history of bleeding from ulcers in his stomach, and has melaena on rectal examination. Which is the single most appropriate immediate management? ★

A Application of a military antishock trouser (MAST) suit

B IV bolus of gelofusine

C IV bolus of 5% dextrose

D IV infusion of noradrenaline (norepinephrine)

E Transfusion of packed red blood cells

9. A 27-year-old man has a sudden onset of severe occipital headache. Which single clinical sign is of greatest concern? ★

A Loss of consciousness

B Neck stiffness

C Photophobia

D Unilateral pain

E Vomiting

10. A 45-year-old man has a systolic blood pressure of 50 mmHg and a pulse rate of 120 bpm. Which single vascular access line would be the best to use? ★

A Green Venflon (18G)

B Grey Venflon (16G)

C Intraosseus needle

D Single-lumen central line

E Triple-lumen central line

11. A 45-year-old scaffolder has fallen 30 feet from a scaffold. He is unconscious and brought in on a spinal board. You wish to 'log roll' him off the spinal board. Which single instruction to the team about a log roll should be given? ★

A A rectal examination must be performed first

B Five members of staff are required in total

C One staff member should take the patient's shoulders and pelvis

D The patient's head must be held slightly flexed on the body

E The staff member who examines the patient's back is in charge

12. A 23-year-old woman has been tackled during a football match and has a fracture of the tibial plateau, which is undisplaced. Which is the single most appropriate method of immobilizing this fracture? ★

A Above-knee back slab

B Below-knee back slab

C Cast brace

D Cricket bat splint

E Wool and crepe bandage

13. A 2-year-old boy is brought to the Emergency Department from his nursery. The nursery staff are concerned because he has multiple bruises on his arms and legs. Which single injury is the most likely to be non-accidental? ★

A Bruising to the anterior shins

B Dislocation of the radial head

C Greenstick fracture of the distal radius

D Hot water splash burns to the arm and face

E Small round bruises on the sides of the chest

14. A 75-year-old man has an acutely red left eye and is vomiting. His visual acuity is 6/24 and he appears very unwell. The eye is red, the cornea is hazy, and the pupil is irregular and unreactive. Which is the single most likely diagnosis? ★

A Acute closed-angle glaucoma

B Central retinal vein thrombosis

C Conjunctivitis

D Episcleritis

E Herpetic ulcer

15. A 34-year-old man is crushed against a wall by a reversing car. He is distressed and has difficulty breathing. Which is the single most reliable sign of a right-sided tension pneumothorax? ★

A Absent breath sounds on the right side

B Dullness of the chest to percussion

C Hyper-resonance to percussion

D The presence of circulatory shock

E Tracheal deviation to the left

16. A 25-year-old man has had a generalized seizure that lasted for 5 minutes. He remains post-ictal and his breathing is noisy. Which single piece of equipment is the most appropriate to use to maintain a patent airway? ★

A Endotracheal tube

B Guedel airway

C Nasopharyngeal airway

D Suction

E Tracheostomy tube

17. A 6-week-old boy has been vomiting immediately after every feed for the last 5 days. He vomits large quantities of non-bilious vomitus, which shoot out all over his mother while she is feeding him. He is screaming hungrily and has sunken eyes and dry mucous membranes. Which is the single most likely diagnosis? ★

A Hirschsprung's disease

B Malrotation of the bowel

C Oesophageal atresia

D Pyloric stenosis

E Urinary tract infection

18. A 54-year-old railway worker is hit by a train. He has an open injury to his right thigh with a fractured femur clearly visible in the wound. There is arterial bleeding from the wound and his systolic blood pressure is 70 mmHg. Which is the single most appropriate immediate action? ★

A Activate the major haemorrhage protocol

B Apply a tourniquet proximally

C Apply pressure to the wound

D Ask the surgeon to cross-clamp the femoral artery

E Explore the wound to clamp the bleeding vessel

19. A 35-year-old man has acute pain in his upper abdomen radiating through to his back, and he is vomiting. Which single factor is most likely to support a diagnosis of pancreatitis? ★

A Contact with gastroenteritis

B Excessive alcohol intake

C History of foreign travel

D History of renal colic

E Use of cocaine and amphetamines

20. A 25-year-old woman has vaginal bleeding. Her husband tells you that they have been undergoing fertility treatment and she is thought to be 2 months pregnant after implantation of fertilized eggs. She has some bleeding from her vagina, with mild left-sided abdominal tenderness. She has a pulse rate of 70 bpm and a systolic blood pressure of 80 mmHg. Which is the single most appropriate action to take in the Emergency Department? ★

A Arrange an urgent ultrasound scan of her pelvis

B Arrange for her to go to theatre

C Give her O-negative blood

D Give her O-positive blood

E Perform a speculum examination

21. A 41-year-old cyclist is brought into the Emergency Department after a collision with a motor vehicle. He appears pale and clammy. His blood pressure is 65/30 mmHg and his heart rate is 145 bpm. He has a grossly hyperexpanded left hemithorax, with tracheal deviation to the right. The neck veins are visibly distended. Which is the single most appropriate initial management? ★

A Bolus 1 L of colloid

B Insert a chest drain

C Perform needle thoracocentesis

D Perform pericardiocentesis

E Transfuse 2 units of O-negative blood

22. A 45-year-old man presents with tachycardia and the ECG shown in Plate 10.1 (see Colour Plate section). Which single feature is thought to be an adverse sign in patients with this condition? ★ ★

A Abdominal pain

B Agitation and confusion

C Systolic blood pressure higher than 180 mmHg

D Redness of the extremities

E Basal crepitations and raised jugular venous pressure

23. A 25-year-old woman has taken 40 paracetamol tablets (20 g). She is refusing to accept medical treatment, stating that she wishes to die. Which is the single most appropriate immediate course of action? ★ ★

A Allow her to go home, as everyone has a right to die

B Assume that she is mentally incompetent and treat her against her wishes

C Contact her GP for more information about her

D Formally assess her capacity to refuse treatment

E Request psychiatry to section her for medical treatment

24. A 95-year-old woman has a leg ulcer on the medial aspect of her lower leg. It is weeping, with necrotic tissue in the centre of the ulcer. After debridement under local anaesthetic, the wound looks pink and has some minor bleeding areas. Which is the single most appropriate dressing to apply? ★ ★

A Alginate dressing

B Flamazine cream

C Iodine-impregnated dressing

D Jelonet® dressing

E Non-adherent dressing

25. A 43-year-old woman is in a coma. Her eyes open to pain, she responds with groans to pain, and she extends to pain. Which is her single Glasgow Coma Scale score? ★ ★

A 3

B 6

C 9

D 12

E 15

26. A 12-year-old boy presents to the Emergency Department following a clash of heads while playing football. Which single aspect of his presentation warrants CT imaging of his head? ★ ★

A He has vomited twice in the Emergency Department

B He has a GCS score of 13

C He has had a seizure in the Emergency Department

D He is bleeding profusely from a forehead laceration

E He reports a pain score of 10/10

27. A 22-year-old male student presents to the Emergency Department after a long train journey. He has noticed non-specific chest pain for the last hour and wanted to get it checked out. He is a non-smoker who is normally well and has no previous medical or significant family history. The ECG is normal. Which single blood test would be useful in this situation? ★ ★

A Coagulation screen

B C-reactive protein

C D-dimer

D Serum amylase

E Troponin I

28. A 68-year-old man is pronounced dead in the Emergency Department after prolonged resuscitation. Which single factor in the history below requires reporting of the death to the coroner/procurator fiscal? ★ ★ ★

A The death is related to a diagnosed terminal illness

B The death is related to travel overseas

C The patient had been in hospital for less than 24 hours

D The patient had seen his GP in the last 2 days

E The patient is not a UK citizen

29. You are walking home from work as a foundation doctor near the railway line when you hear a massive noise. A mainline train has derailed and is lying on its side. There appear to be multiple casualties. Which is the single most appropriate action? ★ ★ ★

A Make your way to the nearest hospital to offer help

B Provide immediate first aid to the nearest casualty

C Telephone 999 and give a formal report

D Telephone the press to give them the news

E Telephone your hospital to let them know

30. An 18-year-old man has been fitting for the last 15 minutes. An oxygen mask is in place and a nasal airway has been inserted by the ambulance crew. One dose of rectal diazepam has been given and a cannula has been inserted. Which is the single most appropriate immediate treatment? ★ ★ ★

A Diazepam 10 mg per rectum

B Lorazepam 4 mg IV

C Midazolam 4 mg IV

D Phenytoin 18 mg/kg IV

E Thiopentone 5 mg/kg IV

31. A 75-year-old diabetic woman has a pre-tibial laceration to her right leg that she sustained 45 minutes ago. She has a barely palpable popliteal pulse and no pulses in the foot. Which is the single most appropriate method of closure? ★ ★ ★ ★

A 30 Ethibond (semi-synthetic) sutures

B 40 Vicryl Rapide sutures

C Primary skin grafting

D Steri-Strips

E Tissue glue

32. A 72-year-old man is acutely short of breath and unwell, his oxygen saturation on air is 75%, and his blood gases show a mildly raised carbon dioxide level and a low oxygen level with a mild mixed acidosis. Which single factor is a contraindication to the use of non-invasive ventilation in this patient? ★ ★ ★ ★

A Epistaxis

B False teeth

C Nausea

D Pneumonia

E Previous respiratory arrest

33. A 75-year-old man has collapsed. He has left-sided facial weakness and a dense left hemiparesis. He is looking towards his right side and appears to have left-sided neglect. There is no obvious visual-field deficit. He has severe dysarthria but no obvious dysphasia. The CT brain scan performed at 6 hours is suggestive of an ischaemic area in the distribution of the right middle cerebral artery. Which single intervention is most likely to optimize his outcome? ★ ★ ★ ★

A Keep his heart rate between 60 and 100 bpm

B Keep his temperature above 37.5°C

C Keep his systolic blood pressure below 100 mmHg

D Maintain his blood glucose level within the normal range

E Maintain his haemoglobin level above 12 g/dL

34. A 78-year-old man is in shock. After initial resuscitation, the decision is made to insert a central line using the subclavian approach. Which is the single most appropriate landmark to give guidance during the procedure? ★ ★ ★ ★

A Insertion is at the junction of the medial and middle thirds of the clavicle

B The clavicle is superior to the subclavian vein

C The needle should be pointing towards the tip of the contralateral scapula

D The subclavian vein lies medial to the subclavian artery

E The subclavian vein runs under the first rib

35. You are asked to act as team leader during the resuscitation of a 30-year-old man. Which is the single most effective behaviour of a team leader? ★ ★ ★ ★

A Check the identity and skills of all team members when they arrive

B Continually ask team members for their opinion

C Insist on silence during the resuscitation unless questioned directly

D Issue all instructions in a loud voice

E Personally perform all invasive procedures

Extended Matching Questions

Causes of chest pain

For each patient with chest pain, choose the *single* most likely diagnosis from the list of options below. Each option may be used once, more than once, or not at all. ★

A Acute coronary syndrome

B Costochondritis

C Myocardial infarction

D Pneumonia

E Pulmonary embolism

F Reflux oesophagitis

G Shingles

H Tuberculosis

1. A 25-year-old woman has had a sharp left-sided chest pain for 4 hours. She fractured her ankle 4 weeks ago when she fell down some stairs on her way outside for a cigarette, and she has been in a plaster cast.

2. A 65-year-old man has had central crushing chest pain and palpitations for 2 hours. An ECG shows new left bundle branch block.

3. A 54-year-old woman has an area on her right chest wall that is excruciatingly painful to touch. There is some redness in a linear distribution over the tender area.

4. A 45-year-old woman has central crushing pain in her chest that wakes her at night and improves on sitting up.

5. A 35-year-old man who is human immunodeficiency virus (HIV)-positive has had right-sided pleuritic chest pain and a productive cough with green sputum for 2 days.

Use of airway adjuncts

For each presentation, choose the *single* most appropriate airway adjunct required from the list of options below. Each option may be used once, more than once, or not at all. ★

A Bag valve mask

B Endotracheal tube

C Guedel airway

D High-flow oxygen with a reservoir mask

E Nasopharyngeal airway

F Surgical airway

G Tracheostomy

H Venturi mask with 24% oxygen

6. A 25-year-old man is recovering from a grand mal seizure, which lasted for 6 minutes and was terminated by a single dose of diazepam.

7. An 85-year-old man with chronic obstructive pulmonary disease (COPD) has a respiratory tract infection and a respiratory rate of 25 breaths/minute.

8. A 56-year-old man has had a serious head and facial injury, and his Glasgow Coma Scale score is 6/15.

9. A 45-year-old woman has been in a house fire and has severe burns around her face, soot in her mouth, stridor, and singed eyebrows.

10. A 10-year-old boy with severe asthma is unable to talk in sentences.

Acute pain relief

For each presentation, choose the *single* most appropriate method of immediate pain relief from the list of options below. Each option may be used once, more than once, or not at all. ★ ★

A Diclofenac 75 mg IM

B Dispersible paracetamol 1 g orally

C Glyceryl trinitrate 1 spray sublingually

D Immediate reduction

E Immobilization with a splint

F Inhaled nitrous oxide

G Morphine 2–10 mg titrated IV

H Oramorph 0.5 mg/kg orally

11. A 56-year-old man has had acute central chest pain for 5 minutes. He is a smoker and has a strong family history of ischaemic heart disease.

12. A 36-year-old man falls from his bicycle and has a dislocated right shoulder. He is in pain and there is a lot of muscle spasm around the shoulder.

13. A 4-year-old boy slips and dislocates the proximal interphalangeal joint of his right little finger.

14. A 25-year-old woman has a high temperature and very painful swollen tonsils.

15. A 35-year-old man has severe right-sided abdominal and loin pain, which is colicky in nature and radiates to his right testis.

Immobilization of fractures

For each presentation, choose the *single* most appropriate method of immobilization from the list of options below. Each option may be used once, more than once, or not at all. ★ ★ ★

A Broad arm sling

B Collar and cuff

C Colles' plaster

D Futura splint

E High arm sling

F Mallet finger splint

G Neighbour strapping

H Scaphoid plaster

16. A 25-year-old man has had an anterior dislocation of his shoulder reduced under IV sedation.

17. An 85-year-old man has a minimally displaced fracture of the surgical neck of his right humerus.

18. A 45-year-old man has pain and crepitus over Lister's tubercle of the right radius, with a normal X-ray.

19. A 25-year-old man has a boxer's fracture of the right fifth metacarpal.

20. A 43-year-old woman has an infected dog bite on the distal phalanx of the left index finger.

ANSWERS

Single Best Answers

1. **A** ★   OHCS 9th edn → p. 798

In any major trauma, cervical spine protection is considered along with the airway. Full protection consists of a rigid collar that is correctly sized, and immobilization with sandbags and tape. Manual in-line immobilization should be used until these are available.

2. **A** ★

This woman has a markedly raised blood sugar level and is acidotic, which indicates diabetic ketoacidosis. After control of airway and breathing, which should always come first, the next priority is to restore circulating volume with a fluid bolus.

3. **C** ★   OHCS 9th edn → p. 632

1–2 mL of 1% lidocaine is sufficient for the majority of wounds. Ring blocks essentially use infiltration of local anaesthetic into the soft tissue around the digital nerve. This results in nerve impulses being blocked before they reach the spinal cord and the cerebral cortex, thus achieving anaesthesia. Two injections are required, one on each side of the finger at the base of the finger. The whole skin of the finger will be anaesthetized by such a block, including the nail bed. There is no greater advantage of 2% lidocaine over 1%, and Emergency Departments are recommended to keep only one strength in stock, in order to minimize the risk of confusion when calculating doses. The use of adrenaline (epinephrine) in any local infiltration around an end artery (the digital artery) is contraindicated because of the risk to perfusion to the distal finger. Other end arteries include the nasal artery and the artery to the penis.

4. **D** ★   OHCS 9th edn → p. 544

This patient is most likely to have developed otitis media in association with her viral upper respiratory tract infection, which has led to a perforation of her eardrum and discharge of pus. It is unlikely that her symptoms are due to a simple otitis externa, as this rarely gives systemic symptoms such as fever in an adult. Although a foreign body may act as a nidus for infection, it is unlikely that the woman's earpiece would have migrated into her ear without being noticed. Wax should not cause systemic upset. An isolated perforation of the eardrum should not cause continued discharge or temperature.

5. B ★   OHCS 9th edn → p. 742

The objective of the immobilization must be considered. This fracture will heal well in time, and there are no strong forces working across the fracture site to displace the fracture. Therefore the key aim of the immobilization is pain relief. A broad arm sling is the most comfortable method of immobilizing the arm, as it provides support for the whole arm and supports the elbow itself. A high arm sling flexes the elbow to over 90° and is therefore uncomfortable in the presence of an elbow effusion. A collar and cuff is used by some, but confers no advantage and allows the elbow to feel the full effects of gravity, which some patients find uncomfortable. A Futura splint (a removable splint that immobilizes the wrist) is not appropriate for the elbow. A back slab is difficult to apply, and if strong enough to keep the elbow from moving will be very heavy. It is not necessary to completely immobilize the joint in this patient.

6. D ★

Erythromycin can inhibit the metabolism of warfarin by affecting the cytochrome P450 complex in the liver, and can therefore enhance its effects.

7. E ★

This is quite common in the elderly, and consideration should be given to ensuring that it does not keep happening. Occupational therapy services can assess the home environment and daily functioning, and can address issues that may predispose to falls.

8. B ★   OHCS 9th edn → p. 726

The priority is fluid resuscitation of the circulating volume. There is an ongoing debate about the use of crystalloid versus colloid solution for this purpose. However, dextrose would not be an appropriate choice of crystalloid solution. Blood would not be given as the primary resuscitation fluid, but may be needed later if there is significant bleeding.

9. A ★

The sudden onset of severe occipital headache suggests a subarachnoid haemorrhage. All of these symptoms may occur in a patient with a subarachnoid haemorrhage, but loss of consciousness suggests rising intracranial pressure and must be treated as an emergency.

10. B ★

This man is significantly shocked and requires fluid resuscitation. A large-bore line is needed, but central lines take too long to insert. Intraosseous needles may be appropriate in young children, but vascular access should be possible in adults.

11. B ★   OHCS 9th edn → p. 774

Five people are required to perform a log roll. One person stands at the patient's head and keeps control of the head, neck, and airway and gives commands, one takes the arms and trunk, one takes the upper legs and pelvis, one supports the calves, and the fifth person examines the back and performs a rectal examination. The patient is rolled gently towards the three supporters of the body and then held in a stable line while the back is examined.

12. A ★   OHCS 9th edn → p. 754

The most important issue in this fracture is to consider what is attached to the fracture site and therefore what the possible displacement or consequences of not immobilizing might be. The tibial plateau is a weight-bearing surface, so any fracture must be treated as non-weight-bearing at first. In addition, the injury pattern often includes injuries to the menisci or collateral ligaments. If the fracture involves the cruciate ligaments (evidenced by involvement of the tibial spine in the fracture line), minimizing the anterioposterior movement of the tibia on the femur is important.

Immobilization techniques must be easy for the patient to manage, and maintain their mobility. Therefore the most appropriate technique for immobilization in the Emergency Department is the above-knee back slab. A below-knee back slab will not restrict the anterioposterior movement of the tibia on the femur. The cast brace is more suitable once the patient has started to mobilize the knee after the initial injury has settled. A cricket bat splint may be useful, as it will allow the patient to wash their leg, but may not be available in the Emergency Department. A wool and crepe bandage was formerly a useful method, but is no longer used because of the extensive resources required and the difficulty for the patient in keeping such a bandage correctly applied.

13. E ★   OHCS 9th edn → p. 146

Accidents are common in toddlers, and it can be difficult to work out which of them are non-accidental. The shins are a very common site for bruising, but the chest, abdomen, and back are not. Small discrete round bruises suggest the use of fingers or an implement. Pulled elbows and greenstick fractures are common in young children, and burns that have splash patterns are more commonly accidental.

14. A ★

This is an ophthalmological emergency, caused by blockage of the flow of aqueous humour from the anterior chamber, which is exacerbated at night when the pupil dilates. It leads to raised intraocular pressure, which causes severe pain, redness, a fixed pupil, and decreased acuity. Drops are required to cause miosis and open the angle.

15. D ★   OHCS 9th edn → p. 724

Tension pneumothorax is an emergency and should be picked up as part of your primary survey in trauma patients. The patient will be in respiratory distress and will be shocked, and tension pneumothorax should always be considered in trauma patients with these features. Other signs are tracheal deviation to the opposite side, hyper-resonance to percussion, and absent breath sounds on that side, but these are unreliable signs.

16. C ★

Patients who are post-ictal may need airway support until they become fully conscious. Guedel (oropharyngeal) airways and suction may trigger a gag reflex. Intubation may be necessary only if the patient does not regain full consciousness within a reasonable time, or if there is further airway compromise for any other reason.

17. D ★

This classically presents at 6 to 8 weeks with projectile milky vomits during or immediately after feeds. There is constipation and the baby seems to be hungry all the time, as he has had no food. A mass may be felt in the midline during a feed, and peristalsis may be seen, but the only reliable way to diagnose pyloric stenosis is with an ultrasound scan.

18. C ★   OHCS 9th edn → pp. 724–725

Following the ABCDE (airway, breathing, circulation, disability, exposure) approach to trauma management, haemorrhage control is part of the assessment and initial management of circulation. This should be done by applying direct pressure on bleeding points in the first instance.

19. B ★

This is the most likely cause of pancreatitis in a young man. Excess alcohol consumption (binge drinking) can cause acute pancreatitis from hours to a couple of days afterwards.

20. E ★   OHCS 9th edn → p. 260

In a miscarriage, products of conception can build up behind the cervical os and cause pressure. The cervix has many stretch receptors, and when it is trying to dilate it can stimulate the vagus nerve, causing haemodynamic instability. This causes bradycardia because of the vagal stimulation, rather than the tachycardia that is seen in severe blood loss. These products need to be removed under direct vision with sponge forceps. Further surgical treatment may be needed, and fluid resuscitation if the blood pressure remains low. An ultrasound scan is the first-line approach in threatened miscarriage, but the haemodynamic instability here makes other options more urgent.

21. C ★

This is a classic presentation of a tension pneumothorax. This life-threatening condition requires immediate needle thoracocentesis—that is, insertion of a wide-bore cannula into the pleural cavity, followed by chest drain insertion. There may also be cardiac tamponade, but this is lower down the list of likely diagnoses based upon the clinical presentation.

22. E ★ ★

This is a broad-complex tachycardia. If the patient is stable, it can be treated with drugs. However, in a patient with signs of heart failure or shock, cardioversion should be performed. Therefore it is important to recognize 'adverse' signs.

23. D ★ ★   OHCS 9th edn → p. 403

The Mental Capacity Act 2005 (England and Wales) states that everyone should be treated as being able to make their own decisions until it has been shown that they cannot. It also aims to enable people to make their own decisions for as long as they are capable of doing so. An individual's capacity to make a decision will be established at the time when a decision needs to be made. A lack of capacity could be due to a severe learning disability, dementia, mental health problems, a brain injury, a stroke, or unconsciousness due to an anaesthetic or a sudden accident. Note that a different Act, the Adults with Incapacity (Scotland) Act 2000, applies in Scotland.

→ www.mentalhealth.org.uk/information/mental-health-a-z/mental-capacity/mental-capacity-act-2005/#incapacityscotland

24. E ★ ★

A non-adherent dressing is recommended after debridement. A current trial is examining the benefit of silver-donating dressings, but currently there is no evidence that these are beneficial. Iodine-impregnated dressings may cause local inflammation and reaction, and are not to be recommended. Alginate dressings have advantages, particularly when the wound has a heavy exudate, but immediately after debridement these should not be necessary.

→ http://cks.library.nhs.uk/leg_ulcer_venous/management/prescribing_information/dressings/choice_of_wound_contact_dressing

25. B ★   OHCS 9th edn → p. 720

The Glasgow Coma Scale score is calculated as follows:

	Score
Best eye response	
No eye opening	1
Eyes open to pain	2
Eyes open to command	3
Eyes open spontaneously	4
Best motor response	
No motor response	1
Extensor posturing to pain	2
Abnormal flexor posturing to pain	3
Withdraws to pain (normal flexion)	4
Localizing response to pain	5
Obeys command	6
Best verbal response	
No sounds	1
Incomprehensible sound	2
Inappropriate speech	3
Confused conversation	4
Normal	5

26. ★ ★ C

National Institute for Health and Clinical Excellence (NICE) guidelines on the management of head injury state that if a post-traumatic seizure occurs, CT imaging of the head is indicated. As this patient is a child, he would need to vomit three times before a scan was indicated, but a single vomit in an adult following head injury would prompt CT scanning.

→ www.nice.org.uk/nicemedia/live/11836/36260/36260.pdf

27. C ★ ★

The D-dimer blood test is only useful if the result is normal, because it can then be used to rule out venous thromboembolism in low-risk patients. D-dimer is a fibrin degradation product which indicates that clotting and subsequent fibrinolysis have been occurring. It is therefore non-specific, and will be raised in many situations (e.g. post-operatively). Local protocols may recommend it in a situation where clinical suspicion of pulmonary embolism (based on risk factors and clinical presentation) is low. The D-dimer test can be performed to enable discharge of the patient with more confidence.

Troponin I is only indicated if there is a suspicion that chest pain may have an ischaemic aetiology. There is nothing to suggest this in this case. The other tests have no role in managing this presentation.

28. C ★ ★ ★

It is important to know which deaths need to be reported to the coroner/procurator fiscal. All deaths that occur within 24 hours of admission must be reported to the coroner's office. The following websites provide guidance:

→ http://www.medicalprotection.org/uk/england-factsheets

→ www.manchester.gov.uk/downloads/download/2185/guidance_notes_for_doctors

29. C ★ ★ ★ OHCS 9th edn → p. 796

Although it may be tempting to help out at major incidents, these are carefully controlled and managed by trained personnel, and your responsibility, even as a doctor, is to allow these teams to take charge, and to act as any other member of the public unless specifically instructed to do otherwise.

30. B ★ ★ ★

There is an established adult Advanced Life Support (ALS) algorithm for the treatment of status epilepticus. First-line treatment consists of benzodiazepines. Diazepam is administered per rectum if there is no access, but lorazepam is preferred once access has been established.

→ www.patient.co.uk/showdoc/40001332/

31. D ★ ★ ★ ★   OHCS 9th edn → pp. 754–755

Pre-tibial lacerations are difficult to heal, even when there is no coexist-ing morbidity. In this patient with both major vessel arterial disease and probable microvascular disease, the blood supply will be severely limited. Any attempt at closure must ensure that the edges are approximated as closely as possible but are not under excessive tension, that there are no foreign bodies in the wound, and that the flap itself is cleaned as thor-oughly as possible. Steri-Strips under as little tension as possible are the most appropriate method of skin closure in this patient. Some minor 'spot welds' of glue might also help to minimize tension while still allowing exudate to leave the wound.

Vicryl Rapide is a dissolving suture (after 7–10 days) that is suitable for subcutaneous sutures, but it is not appropriate for this wound, for which the healing time may be up to 6 weeks. Ethibond can be used to close wounds, but would be too heavy and would lead to tissue strangulation between the sutures. Although a proportion of pre-tibial lacerations result in skin grafting, primary grafting is not recommended because of the risk associated with anaesthetic and the creation of a second wound, particularly in a high-risk patient, such as this diabetic woman with arteriopathy.

→ www.cks.nhs.uk/lacerations#

32. A ★ ★ ★ ★

33. D ★ ★ ★ ★

Hyperglycaemia after stroke worsens brain injury. Large randomized controlled trials have shown that keeping blood sugar levels within tight limits leads to better outcomes.

Gentile NT, Seftchick MW, Huynh T, Kruus LK, and Gaughan J (2006). Decreased mortality by normalizing blood glucose after acute ischemic stroke. *Acad Emerg Med* **13:** 174–180.

34. B ★ ★ ★ ★

→ www.surgical-tutor.org.uk/default-home.htm

35. A ★ ★ ★ ★

Extended Matching Questions

1. E ★

Immobility and smoking are risk factors for pulmonary embolism in this patient.

2. C ★

Central crushing chest pain always raises the suspicion of myocardial infarction. Although the ECG changes are not classic ST elevation, new bundle branch block is also indicative of ischaemia.

3. G ★

The pain of shingles (herpes zoster) can be excruciating, but is localized to a dermatomal distribution. The typical vesicular rash is not always present first.

4. F ★

Reflux is often position dependent, so is worse when lying or bending down, because of gravity.

5. D ★

In immunocompromised patients there is an increased risk of pneumonia. The cough with green sputum, even in the absence of fever, is indicative.

6. E ★

7. H ★

8. B ★

9. F ★

10. D ★

General feedback on 6–10: Airway interventions range from basic (Guedel airway) to advanced. Patients should be managed with the most basic intervention, except in cases where it is obvious that advanced airway skills will be needed— that is, unconscious patients or those in whom there is likely to be difficulty in maintaining the airway over time (e.g. due to airway burns). The oxygen concentration delivered should initially be as near to 100% as possible, except in those situations where it is likely that the patient is relying upon hypoxic drive for breathing (e.g. patients with chronic obstructive pulmonary disease).

11. C ★ ★

This is a picture of angina, and glyceryl trinitrate spray will relieve the pain by acting as a general and coronary vasodilator.

12. G ★ ★

Although the other methods will achieve pain relief, morphine will also relax the muscles to enable reduction. Nitrous oxide may be used, but will be hard to hold and will take longer to become effective.

13. D ★ ★

This is easy to reduce, and if done immediately will cause rapid pain relief. If it can be performed straight away, time should not be wasted waiting for analgesia to be administered.

14. B ★ ★

Paracetamol is an antipyretic and provides effective pain relief for minor illnesses.

15. A ★ ★

This is renal colic, and non-steroidal anti-inflammatory drugs will provide effective pain relief. If given by the intramuscular route, they act quickly.

General feedback on 11–15: OHCS 9th edn → pp. 636, 802

16. A ★ ★ ★

17. B ★ ★ ★

18. D ★ ★ ★

19. G ★ ★ ★

20. E ★ ★ ★

General feedback on 16–20: Injuries to the shoulder joint or clavicle should be immobilized in a broad arm sling to enable the sling to take the weight of the limb and thus relieve pain. An anterior dislocation of the shoulder is best treated in a broad arm sling, with or without a body bandage, to keep the arm adducted and in internal rotation, thus avoiding the dislocating movement. Fractures to the humeral shaft, starting at the surgical neck, require a collar and cuff to allow the weight of the arm to reduce the fracture and maintain anatomical alignment. It is difficult to immobilize a proximal fracture of the humerus in plaster, because of the anatomy of the axilla.

The Futura splint is useful for immobilization, as the wearer can remove the splint for personal care and gentle mobilization. Tenosynovitis responds well to immobilization and non-steroidal anti-inflammatory drugs.

Any injury to the fingers or metacarpals is best treated with minimal immobilization, to allow the hand to continue to function. Neighbour strapping encourages the injured digit to move, but minimizes the strain on the injured part. The ligaments around the small joints of the hand are prone to fibrosis and shortening. Therefore gentle mobilization is essential to prevent long-term contractures and loss of function.

Any infection or injury that has resulted in extensive swelling of the digits should be managed with a high arm sling. The high arm sling is designed to maintain the hand at the level of the shoulder, whereas the broad arm sling maintains the hand at the level of the elbow. Simple elevation is key to the management of most hand injuries, and should be adopted for at least the first 48 hours.

Index

Note: Page numbers in *italics* denote answers